Relating to the Relatives

breaking bad news, communication and support

with Margaret Spalding

Radcliffe Medical Press
Oxford and New York

© 1996 Thurstan Brewin with Margaret Sparshott

Radcliffe Medical Press Ltd
18 Marcham Road, Abingdon, Oxon OX14 1AA, UK

Radcliffe Medical Press, Inc.
141 Fifth Avenue, New York, NY 10010, USA

British Library Cataloguing in Publication Data

A catalogue record for this book is available from the British Library.

ISBN 1 85775 081 0

Library of Congress Cataloging-in-Publication Data is available.

Typeset by TechType, Abingdon, Oxon
Printed and bound by Biddles Ltd, Guildford and King's Lynn

Thurstan Brewin is a Fellow of The Royal College of Physicians. Since retirement from his post as a consultant in Clinical Oncology in Glasgow, he has worked with three medical charities – Marie Curie Cancer Care, the Sue Ryder Foundation and HealthWatch.

Margaret Sparshott is a trained nurse of many years' experience, now retired but still continuing to work on an 'as and when' basis in the Neonatal Intensive Care Unit of Derriford Hospital, Plymouth. She is the author of many articles on the environmental problems of the newborn, and also lectures on the subject. In 1991 she won the NT/3M National Nursing Award for practice, for her contribution towards reducing infant trauma.

One of the best pieces of advice ever given to doctors, nurses or other health workers is that each time they see a patient they ask themselves two questions:

- What can I do for this patient?
- What can I learn from this patient?

The same applies when seeing relatives:

- What can I *do for* this relative?
- What can I *learn from* this relative?

There is always something to do – and always something to learn.

Always.

Contents

Acknowledgements

My grateful thanks to Margaret Sparshott, not only for writing the chapter about helping relatives of sick children – and for sharing the writing of the chapter on the angry relative – but for checking what I have written in the rest of the book and for many helpful suggestions.

Second, I cannot adequately express my thanks to those many hospital colleagues, family doctors, nursing staff, social workers and others with whom I have had helpful discussions over the years, nor to countless relatives in England, Scotland and Canada for what they have taught me. And especially for letting me know when I have said the wrong thing, or failed to say the right thing. This is how you learn.

Introduction

Who is this book intended for?

It is intended for all those who not only have to give bad news, but who are also keen to give as much help and support as possible to partners and families – both immediately and during remission, relapse, terminal illness, dying or grieving.

Note: 'Relatives' – the general word used for convenience by most doctors and nurses (in the absence of anything better) – is used throughout to include *anyone* close to the patient: a wife or husband, an unmarried partner (not necessarily of the opposite sex), an adult son or daughter, a parent or any close friend or member of the family.

Time is like money. More of it spent on one thing means less for other things. Five minutes more with relatives may mean five minutes less with patients. The doctor who wants to help relatives doesn't want to be thought of as neglecting patients. How do we decide on priorities?

Here is one physician who wished he had given relatives a higher priority: 'Were I to be in charge of wards again', wrote Sir Derrick Dunlop (looking back on his career and wondering how he might do better if given a second chance), 'I would try to be present more often at visiting times to answer the questions of anxious relatives.'[1]

'Talking to the relatives is essential for the welfare of the patient and his friends... it is an art not to be despised', wrote Hugh Barber, who also described more than 50 years ago how a colleague, when interviewing a prospective assistant for his practice, would ask, 'Can you talk to the relatives? That's what matters.'

Perhaps we underestimate the importance of this particular side of the practice of medicine. Good communication with patients must always come first. Nothing could be more important but in various situations and in various stages of an illness, good communication with those nearest to the patient not only gives them information, it is also a powerful way of giving them courage and confidence.

And by helping them we help the patient. For example, a word of encouragement or reassurance – intended for patients, but spoken to relatives and then passed on by them to patients – may sometimes have more effect than when the same thing is said directly to patients. Perhaps it carries more conviction.

Equally, patients will sometimes tell relatives things that they would not tell staff (for example about side-effects – because they don't want to seem cowardly or ungrateful), and this is one of many areas in which the relatives can teach us and help us. The wise doctor stays in touch with them.

In these days of increasing litigation it's impossible to ignore another reason for being on friendly terms with partners and relatives – for supporting them and explaining to them all the difficulties of a serious situation. If things go badly – and the patient gets worse when it had been hoped he would improve – a good relationship will make it much less likely that relatives will feel bitter, suspicious or hostile without good cause.

Note also that although this book concentrates on the somewhat neglected interests of relatives, much of it is very relevant to patients. This is for three main reasons.

- Many general communication skills are discussed.

- Relatives in the role of carer often wish to discuss with a doctor or nurse how they can best communicate with the patient and provide support.

- Relatives are to some extent victims, not just carers, so we sometimes need to approach them in much the same way that we approach patients.

Perhaps this relevance to *patients* in a book addressed to the problems of *relatives* will be seen not just as inevitable, but as an advantage. Seeing the problems of patients through the eyes of those nearest to them may inject new blood into a subject much written about in recent years, but perhaps not from quite this angle.

My experience is more with the relatives of cancer patients than with others, but – aside from the shattering emotional impact of the word cancer – the problems are often much the same. And though I've spent far more time in the hospital environment than in primary care, I hope that these pages may be of some relevance to work in both disciplines – indeed to all those who have any contact with the relatives of the seriously ill whether doctors, nurses, social workers, administrators, spiritual advisers or others. Perhaps they will find something of value in it when they are still in training; perhaps in the early years after qualification.

> **Note: The contribution of the main author is based chiefly on personal experience between 1950 and 1990. Over many years I made occasional notes on this subject at the end of a day, recording on scraps of paper practical lessons learned or perhaps just the comments of relatives. I then filed them away and have used them in this book.**

Some attitudes have changed during this 40-year period, especially with regard to the spelling out of every risk and every grim diagnosis and prognosis. Yet the actual practice has changed less than the rhetoric. Though doctors and nurses, like judges in a court of law, must not just go their own way, they need to retain their instinct for common sense and not be pushed too far by slogans of an unrealistic kind. Since there can never be a complete solution to this dilemma, the pendulum is bound to swing back and forth.

This book tries to bridge the gap – to be sensitive, yet realistic – aiming to mix the best of the old with the best of the new.

When writing for a mixed readership – some far more experienced than others – there is a constant danger of sounding dogmatic or patronizing. Some readers may feel that in no way do they need me to suggest things of which they are already well aware, or are a matter of personal taste. I can only plead that this thought frequently occurred to me; and more than once nearly led to abandoning the whole idea.

Reference

1   Dunlop D (1977) Fifty years on. *World Medicine*. 21 Sep.: 112–13.

Prologue

Doctor: ... *so we can't promise to cure your mother, but there is at least a very fair chance that we can ...*

Relative: *I'm sorry, but you seem to be saying two opposite things. I want to know whether my mother can be cured or not. Please just tell me the truth. If you can't cure her, just say so. I think I have a right to know, I'm her son.*

Doctor: *If I knew, I'd tell you. You want the facts. I understand that. So would I if I were in your position. Well the facts are these. It's a 50 : 50 situation. In other words about half the women of your mother's age and in the situation that she is now in sooner or later die of their disease; and half live a normal life and ultimately die of something else, as we must all do one day.*

Relative: *But you surely must have some idea which half she is in.*

Doctor: *No. I'm afraid not. We truly don't know. If I thought that in your mother's case the outlook was better than 50:50 I'd tell you. And if I thought it was worse than 50:50 I'd tell you. Don't forget that every woman of your mother's age, however healthy, however good for her age, knows that she may not live more than another five or ten years. She may, but she may not. It's not just ill people who face uncertainty. We all do.*

Relative: *I suppose that's right. But it's still a terrible shock. Why should this happen to her? She's done nothing to deserve it.*

Doctor: *No, of course not. It could happen to anyone. The same thing could have happened in my family. It isn't anyone's fault. I've told her that she now has to live with a bit more uncertainty than she lived with before. She could have a recurrence, but we are hoping that she won't. No promises, but real, genuine hope that she will do well.*

Relative: *I'm confused. I just don't know now what to think.*

Doctor: *You find the uncertainty frustrating. I can understand that. But I'm afraid you are going to have to live with it, just as your mother will have to. Sorry, but that's life. You have a choice now between either being optimistic or pessimistic. You can either hope for the best – or you can expect the worse and be especially pleased if she does well. The facts make it quite reasonable for you to look at it in either of these ways. How you look at it is up to you. But don't you think that your mother would prefer to get back to a normal life and be as optimistic as possible? My impression is that she is that sort of person and I think you should join her and be the same. Do you understand what I'm saying?*

Relative *(still looking unhappy)*: *I suppose so, so long as you are not holding anything back ...*

Doctor: *I promise you I'm not.*

Relative: *OK, then ... thanks.*

Five minutes later he is talking on the 'phone to his sister:

All the doctor would say is that she might be cured and she might not. It was very unsatisfactory. He just refused to say any more than that – and now I don't know where we are. Maybe he knows it's going to come back, but just didn't like to say so ...

Surgeon *(to patient's daughter)* : *Your mother's situation is very serious, but it's not hopeless. I promise you that. If the tests we are doing are OK, we can operate and this gives her a chance. We have had patients in this situation who have done well. Unfortunately, there have only been a few of them. But major surgery for elderly people is much safer these days than it used to be, and we naturally want to give everyone the same chance if they are fit enough – the same small chance of doing well. Do you agree that we give your mother that chance?*

Relative *(who has got something all ready to say, so hasn't been listening properly)*: *Doctor, we have talked this over in the family and what we feel is that if the treatment is not going to do any good; we don't want her to have it. I know that as a doctor you are not allowed to give up, but that's how we feel.*

Surgeon: *I understand how you feel, but it's not quite like that. I can assure you that we are not tied by any rules of that kind. If we knew for sure that it wouldn't do any good, we wouldn't do it. If it was my own mother who was in the same situation, my first feelings might well be the same as yours. But I'd like you to think carefully about it, because surgery gives her a chance. And we don't think she has any chance without it.*

A few patients in this situation do really well, but only a few. Do you want your mother to have a chance of doing well, even though it's only a small chance? Or do you hate the thought of making a decision like that? I agree it's difficult ... do you think we should put it to your mother and see what she says?

Relative: *Oh no, doctor, I really don't think we should do that, do you? I mean, she gets quite muddled sometimes. I just don't think she could cope with a decision like that. Especially as, like so many of her generation, she just assumes that doctors and nurses know the best thing to do.*

Surgeon: *Very well then. We are doing some tests and we've got a day or two before we need to decide, so how about you going back to the family and tell them what I said. And just one thing ... before you go, do you mind my asking you what you will tell them that I said?*

Relative: *Well ... I'll tell them that you seem to understand how we feel ... and that you wouldn't do it, if you didn't think it would do any good ...*

Surgeon: *That's more or less it. The only thing that's not quite right is the idea that if it wasn't going to do any good, we wouldn't do it. The point is that it might be successful, but unfortunately it's more likely to fail. That's the* *trouble. We have two choices. Either we say that since it would* probably *not do any good, we are not going to do it. Or we say that we want her to be given a chance,* because it's her only chance – *and because a* few *people who have had this operation have responded well.*

Relative: *We just don't want her to have it if it's not going to do any good.*

Surgeon *(assessing this relative and deciding not to make any further attempt to explain to her that it's not as easy as that)*: *I understand ... I tell you what ... while you are talking with other members of your family, shall I have a word with the nurses and see what they think? Would you like me to do that? They've got to know your mother quite well now. And they'll have the best idea of what it's like for patients to go through this operation and how much distress and discomfort it involves. They might even gently try talking to her a little about it. Then we'll meet again and come to a decision.*

Relative: *Very well.*

Surgeon: *One more question. Has you mother ever expressed a view on the best thing when people her age find themselves in this sort of situation? What I mean is, does she think people ought to seize every chance? Or would she rather let things take their course and just have the best possible care and attention, but without any surgery (surgery that would be followed by tubes and drips and intensive care and all that sort of thing)?*

Relative: *Well, doctor, she's a great fighter, and I wouldn't like you to think she wasn't. But she was saying the other day she reckons that on the whole she's had a good life and she's not complaining. That sounds a bit like she wouldn't want to go through a lot more, doesn't it?*

Surgeon: *I agree, it does.*

Relative: *That's what I meant at the beginning, doctor, we don't want to go against your advice, but if it's not going to do any good, we'd all really rather she didn't go through with it.*

Surgeon: *OK then. How about you 'phoning me tomorrow evening at this number and we'll come to a decision.*

Relative: *Thank you, I'll do that.*

Surgeon *(two days later to the youngest doctor in the team)*: *Did you get the message about Mary Black? I've talked to her daughter and, though she is pretty upset that the family can't seem to agree – and she herself finds it* *difficult to think straight on the subject – they certainly don't want any fur-ther attempts made to find out exactly what her mother wants. Nor do the nurses; they don't think she could cope with any more questions like that. The fact is she is very weary of hospitals and would just love to be back in her own home. So her daughter and I both tend to feel that, on balance, we should give up any idea of surgery.*

Young doctor: *But I thought we had agreed that if the lab. tests and the scans were OK, then surgery would be something that we really ought to do – that it wouldn't be right just to give up. Shall I say the patient has refused – or that the family has refused?*

Surgeon: *Neither. I don't like either of those ways of putting it. Put it down as a joint decision after talking with the family. That'll be best. It's difficult – but let's not ask for any more opinions. There's not going to be any surgery and she can go home.*

Young doctor: *Is that final, then?*

Surgeon: *Yes, I think we have all talked enough. You weren't here yesterday, otherwise I'd like to have had you in on the discussion. She's not for surgery and she can go home ... I think she'll be relieved ...*

Note: The above dialogues are fictitious and were written to illus-trate common problems with no easy answer. All others in the book are either exact quotes or are closely based on actual situations doc-umented at the time.

Who will see the relatives?

On hospital ward rounds the traditional question (after all other aspects of a serious newly diagnosed case have been discussed) has been 'And who will see the relatives?' Or sometimes just 'Who will tell the relatives?' As if 'telling' was all there was to it, a one-way interview in which the relative is seen only as a receiver of bad news, a sort of passive receptacle, merely to be dealt with as kindly as possible.

But if we are to follow the golden rule (putting ourselves in the place of the relative), we must do better than that. There needs to be a two-way conversation of the kind that we'd hope for if we were the relative or partner of a seriously ill person.

So it's never merely 'Who will see this man's wife and give her the bad news?' It's more:

- Who will explain the situation to her and answer her questions?

- Who will give her a chance to get to know us better? And hopefully let her see that we understand how she feels – and that what we want for the patient is the same as what she wants.

- Who will seek her help and hear her views about the patient and his ill-ness?

- Who will enrol her as a vital member of the caring team and start to give her some practical advice and training?

- Who will see if she has any groundless fears or feelings of guilt? Who will give her confidence, moral support and encouragement?

- Who will make a preliminary assessment of the home situation?

Which is a lot of questions. And, of course, there isn't always either the time or the need to consider all of them. But at least such a list emphasizes that a patient's partner or relative should never be regarded as just a receiver of information, but as:

- a receiver of information
- a provider of information
- an adviser
- a carer
- a victim.

At times all these roles are equally important. At other times one is strongly predominant. But even in the briefest interview it's best to give at least a moment's thought to all of them. This is the secret of successfully 'seeing the relatives'.

The legal position: In law the partner or next of kin has no right to information unless the patient has expressly authorized it (or is not sufficiently mentally competent to do so). Some doctors are reluctant to depart from this strict legal position, but most will agree that this is one of those areas where custom and common sense often dictate otherwise. Whenever a patient is in hospital, or ill in their own home, most anxious and caring next of kin will feel quite strongly that they have an immediate right to know what's going on and how serious the position is, whether or not the patient's permission has been formally obtained. Apart from anything else to refuse to say anything could cause them great anxiety.

It may be a little different in an outpatient clinic.

In any serious situation the wise doctor, nurse or social worker will want to *assess* each relative – both as a potential carer and as a potential sufferer and victim. Has she had experience of similar situations? What seem to be her psychological state and her physical health and strength?

Ideally, the hospital doctor would always discuss such things with the family doctor. If they can do so, both will benefit, especially the specialist. But all too often neither can find the time for it.

So it's all quite complex, and there seldom seems to be enough time to deal adequately with every aspect mentioned or with every way in which we might be of help. This contrasts with the remark of a colleague who once asked me, when he saw that I was speaking on this subject, 'How will you fill 25 minutes talking about the patient's relatives?'

Teaching and learning

Perhaps my colleague meant that many insights and strategies in the field of communication come mainly from experience and are almost too subtle to teach. If so, I have a certain sympathy with this traditional view. Good communication, whether with patients or relatives, comes naturally to some people, though there is always room for improvement. For various reasons others find it much harder. To a considerable extent, no matter how well taught, it must always be dependent on personality, on ingrained empathy and on an innate approach to illness and distress that ought to help entry to medical school.

So why not two or three weeks of compulsory unpaid hospital work for all aspiring medical students to observe how they get on with patients and their anxious relatives? It should surely count for something whenever competing applicants are of similar academic standing.

However, recent work by Maguire and others suggests that, even though this is undeniably a very different matter from the teaching of, say, anatomy or biochemistry, real improvement can result from new teaching techniques.[1] Perhaps in groups, discussing a video of how the trainee performs when interviewing either an actor or an actual patient or relative.

Advice may be given by specialists in the art of communication. Or by those with the greatest experience of giving bad news. Ask the nursing staff which doctors do it best; they know. But those who teach must also be willing and able to discuss with others how they have learned from their mistakes; and this doesn't always follow.

When trying to teach this subject there is an interesting problem. Most students, who will avidly write down biochemical or similar hard data given to them, will immediately stop taking notes when offered advice about talking to anxious relatives.

Yet such advice is no more than the offering of approaches to *try* in different situations. Some of the things suggested will suit the personality of some doctors and nurses, but not that of others. Each needs to try them for himself or herself. And they must constantly seek the feedback that will tell them the effect on the relative of what they have said.

Learning by example

Learning by example gets less mention these days. But much can be learned just from being with someone who has plenty of experience of talking to relatives – and who does it well. Don't forget that some of those who are best at it would have great difficulty giving a lecture on the subject.

This doesn't mean that you copy slavishly everything you hear said or see done; however good the person setting an example, only an unthinking zombie would do that. Apart from the fact that nobody gets it right every time, it's not only patients and relatives who vary. Doctors do, too.

Moreover a student can actually learn from watching *poor* communication *badly* done. You note the ineffectiveness or the harm – and you vow that when it comes to your turn you will not so easily omit what *should* have been said, nor say (or at least not say so clumsily) what you feel would have been better left *unsaid*.

Finally, relatives themselves, though they may not know it, are always teaching us something. Not just some relatives, but all of them, for no two relatives and no two situations are ever exactly alike. And if we approach our work in the right way, we never stop learning from them.

Concise communication

All students should be taught by example and discussion that there is an art in warm, effective, *concise* communication, making the best use of every minute. Some talks and articles in recent years have contained almost as much rhetoric as practical advice – 'time must be found for as much listening and counselling as each patient and relative needs, because this is their right' – that sort of thing is not very helpful when it comes to deciding on priorities when under pressure.

Moreover it may encourage the idea that roughly the same amount of time must be given to every patient and relative with similar problems. Or that the amount of time should be symbolic of the seriousness of the situation. Both these ideas can be wasteful and can in the real world deny attention to those who need it most. Korsch and her colleagues found no correlation between satisfaction with an interview and its length.[2]

And even if a doctor or nurse has all the time in the world:

- some relatives *prefer* a brisk business-like approach, with a minimum of chat

- some may *resent* any enquiry about their personal problems

- there is always a risk that mentioning something that the relative was not worrying about (until now) will trigger *new fears*.

The idea that a long session is essential may also encourage some doctors to opt out completely. They refer a patient for specialized advice and coun- selling (for which there may be a waiting list) in situations where a few minutes of warm and positive communication might transform the situation and provide – without any delay – all that is needed. And if what is said in a few minutes is not quite everything that might be said in an ideal world, then at least anything more should have a fairly low priority when under pressure to meet the needs of patients or of other relatives.

As stressed in other parts of this book, for those who are not blind to the essential elements of feedback, it is often written all over a person's face – either that they are already well pleased and encouraged with what has been said, or that more listening and advice are required.

Nothing suggested in this book is suitable every time. They are only things to try. Even when very doubtful about a suggestion, or if you are at a stage in your career when you don't have a lot of experience and have never tried this particular approach, why not make a note to try it some time? Then judge (from both immediate and later feedback) whether or not it has, in your hands, helped and informed the relative in the way you hoped it would.

Getting started

- So far as possible always grasp the essential facts of each case before, not after, the relative enters. Personal data – age, job, family – not just medical data. A good memory for detail is a priceless asset for a doctor. Nothing kills empathy so much as reading case notes in front of the per- son you are interviewing. When this is unavoidable be sure to ask for permission and apologize for having to do it.

- In serious illness it is even more important than usual to stand up imme- diately relatives enter the room and, if possible, take a step or two towards them. Don't just let them come to you. Be glad to see them. Move towards them. Perhaps thank them for coming to see you. Don't let them get the feeling that they are an unwelcome intrusion. This is not just a matter of courtesy; it shows that you accept the challenge of serious situations and that you are not afraid to face them.

- It goes without saying that, if doctor and relative have not met before, an important part of what should be normal courtesy is for the doctor to introduce herself and give the relative her name. In the hospital environment many relatives these days will also want to know the *status* of the person they are seeing and their position in the team, and this should be made plain.

- As you take their arm or shake their hand (but be sensitive; some may prefer you not to) steer them to a seat. Address them by whatever name and style you guess they will prefer, but it's probably best when meeting for the first time – especially if the relative is elderly – to be fairly formal.

- Even when the situation to be discussed is grim, a slight but warm smile of understanding will nearly always be appreciated. Anything less is liable to make you seem cold and remote.

Then (not always, but frequently) a quick word about something quite mundane and normal – the weather, or an item in the news that everyone is talking about, or the difficulty of finding somewhere to park a car, something like that. *Almost* in a totally relaxed, natural way, as if there were nothing very important on the agenda. But not quite. There should be just a hint of the gravity of what needs to be discussed.

How can such trivial small talk be appropriate in a serious situation? I have even seen it claimed that this is a common failing of doctors, and that it is never appropriate. But anyone who says this can have little experience of the surprisingly powerful benefit that often follows if it's done *in the right way*. Presumably because it cuts down fear and tension by its friendly normality, puts the relative more at her ease and reduces fear. And because it shows that the doctor is human.

But, like everything else suggested in this book, if done the wrong way it can be useless or even harmful. One mistake, for example, would be to take too long over it. This could suggest an insensitive failure to appreciate that the relative's mind is in turmoil, wondering what is going to be said. Or it could mean an overall awkwardness and embarrassment. Or, worse still, a wish to postpone for as long as possible the serious things that sooner or later have to be said.

Now *sit down* with the relative. Not directly opposite (which is too formal), nor side by side (which is too informal), but something between the two. And sit within touching distance, so that either of you can touch the other should you wish to at any time.

- It's often best to start with *something crisp and definite about the immediate future* and what the plan is for the next few days (or the next week or two, whichever is appropriate).

- Especially when meeting a relative for the first time, don't forget that the first thing said is often the best remembered – and sometimes the only thing remembered. So don't be tied down by such logical sequences as always saying what has been found before saying how serious it is – *sometimes reverse the order.*

Empathy and understanding

If the doctor is to start off on the right foot when switching from brief preliminary courtesies and small talk to the real problem, it is essential not only to be serious, but also to *look* serious and concerned, so that the relative immediately feels that the doctor has at least some idea of the hell of fear and doubt and anxiety that she may be going through.

Just to *look* as if you understand is a help, provided you don't look *too* concerned or *too* sad, because – as all good doctors and nurses know (and all good friends for that matter) – this can suggest weakness, rather than positive help and strength.

For any doctor or other health worker with any imagination, it shouldn't be difficult – quite apart from whether or not they have had personal experience of similar situations – for the concern shown to be sincere. There is only one rule of medical practice, said Joseph Lister a hundred years ago: put yourself in the patient's place. This should apply just as much to relatives: put yourself in the relative's place.

If relatives get the impression you are doing this, it can provide strong moral support. In addition it suggests that, at least as far as you are concerned, everything done or not done, whether tests or treatment, will be solidly based on concern for the patient and full recognition of his or her special needs, sensibly blended with what you would like for yourself or a member of your family in a similar situation. The hopes of loving relatives are your hopes. Their fears are your fears.

In recent years studies on both sides of the Atlantic have suggested that this sort of concern may be very evident in medical students when they start in medical school, and then becomes, much weaker when they become young doctors a few years later. I have not myself seen this happen. In my experience the man or woman who starts as a caring and concerned person when talking to patients or relatives broadly remains so, however much technical skill and specialized knowledge they subsequently acquire. But perhaps something is now happening that I've missed – possibly connected with the increased stress and pressure put upon junior doctors, owing to such factors as less trust, more new cases admitted each week, more lengthy explaining, more paperwork, more fear of litigation and so on.

Friendly professional interest

With relatives, as with patients, both initially and throughout subsequent contacts and interviews, there is an overriding need for what I have called FPI – friendly professional interest. Relatives, too, need friendship. Relatives, too, need understanding.

- The doctor or nurse should be natural, warm and **friendly**. Sensing, as good friends do, when to talk and when to be silent, when to joke and when to be serious. A sudden *spontaneous* comment of the sort that is clearly not part of any learned technique or preconceived plan can be very valuable, even when giving bad news, partly because it is essentially natural, *friendly* and sincere.

  The friendship offered by professionals is not quite the same as that offered by friends or neighbours. As with leadership, it's often best to keep something back and not to become *too* familiar. But it's sometimes very close to it.

- Second, even if the outlook is 'hopeless', what is said to the relative should reflect the fact that the approach to the patient's problems remains *positive* and **professional**. For example, however certain the main diagnosis and however poor the outlook, not every symptom is due to the main diagnosis. Far from it. Many relatives will have more confidence in a doctor who discusses such points with them, however briefly. This can make a real contribution to the peace of mind of both patient and partner.

- Finally, turning to the third part of FPI, it should quickly become clear to the relative that the doctor is sincerely **interested** in two things:

  - the patient's symptoms and problems, how she is feeling from day to day, how she is sleeping and so on.

  - the patient's life story and life-style. And perhaps in that of the relative, too. No matter how busy the doctor, or how bad the prognosis, or how old or helpless the patient, this interest must be clearly expressed (a few words may be enough). This not only helps the person being spoken to, but also broadens the doctor's understanding and increases the interest and satisfaction of what is in so many ways the best job in the world.

At the same time, as already mentioned, don't forget that some people don't want to discuss their private life and personal problems with anyone and may resent any attempt to do so. This must be instantly recognized and respected. And full advantage taken of it, for it means more time to give to others.

But, like so many other things discussed in this book, remember also that this situation may change. Watch out for clues to the fact that the person who didn't want a conversation of this kind a month ago may now be glad of it.

Relative: *I don't know if you can understand this, doctor, but in a way I want to know exactly how serious my wife's condition is and in a way I'd rather not know.*

- Throughout every interview, short or long, every effort must be made to appear relaxed and unhurried, giving full and undivided attention to the situation and switching off all other concerns, even when under great pressure.

- Fortunately, there are still many patients and relatives who can be greatly helped in a fairly brief, concise way. Indeed they may have no wish for more, even in a serious situation. Especially when they see the needs of others.

- At the end of the interview, always thank relatives for their help, preferably specifying particular points they have made that you have found helpful.

- Then finish with the same kind of brief, friendly, 'irrelevant', non-medical comment that put them at their ease when they arrived, and usually accompany this with a handshake.

Doctor to patient: *Didn't your wife tell you what we talked about? Well, let's see, we talked about how you first met; and what a difficult man you can be sometimes; and how you once forgot to collect one of your children from school.*

Patient (smiling): *She told you that story? That's not fair. Wait 'till I see her!*

Doctor: *Seriously, we had a good talk about you. The fact is she's pretty worried. And the reason is she's so fond of you. You are a lucky man to have a wife like that.*

Patient: *I know doctor, I know. It's more than I deserve. Is my outlook pretty hopeless, then? I mean, how long have I got?*

Doctor (in a friendly, understanding way and with a gentle smile that must be sincere and never of a patronizing kind): *Hang on a minute. I know how you feel, but it would be crazy to jump to conclusions like that before we've even completed the tests. Listen. What I suggest, if you agree, is this. The first thing is to see what this week's tests show. The additional information we get from them will help to plan your treatment. Then next week the three of us meet together to review the situation and talk things over. After that a lot may depend on how well you respond to any treatment we may try.*

Good communication must be *realistic*

Many things affect both understanding and the ability to recall what was said. An important practical point is that the first thing said is often the best remembered. The more anxious or shocked the listener, the more true this is and the simpler the message needs to be. Short words and phrases are usually best, so long as they don't sound patronizing.

When misquoting or misunderstanding occur, the first cause to consider is that the doctor has communicated badly, has been seriously inadequate in some way or has ignored such basic principles as those given on the preceding pages. But it sometimes happens that there was nothing basically wrong with what was said or how it was said; other staff present will confirm this. The misunderstanding was hardly, if at all, the doctor's fault.

What is wanted, when there is a general debate or discussion of this problem of misconceptions and how they arise, is cool and realistic pooling of the experiences of health staff.

- *Shock* is one reason for the relative not taking in even the most basic part of the message, never mind the detail.

- Another is when his mind is so filled with *his own theories and beliefs* that there is no room for anything else.

In both cases the anxious relative may sometimes ask question after question, but not listen properly to any of the answers.

When two relatives are asked what a previous doctor told them, they will often disagree, even though they were together at the time. This is an indication of how common it is for relatives to misunderstand or misquote what was said.

As discussed in Chapter 4 all health staff should be especially wary about accepting at face value what they are told another member of staff said to a patient or relative. A request for more details of what was said may sometimes be all that is needed to reveal something very different from the first version.

Is this problem of misconception ever a valid reason for making what is said as short and straightforward as possible? In the real world, yes, without any doubt. But this must never be done lightly.

Other reasons why it may occasionally seem wise to keep what is said to the essential minimum are:

- the relative may trust the doctor to do her best, is weary of explanations and just wants the patient to start treatment

- the doctor's personality is more suited to the role of being 'strong and silent' than it is to explaining everything – except where really necessary

- old age, confusion, deafness, short attention span, etc. mean that the relative can only grasp one or *at the most two* simple messages

- pressure of work, other relatives waiting to be seen and other priorities mean that there is no time for details, only for simple basic messages.

Reducing the risk of misconception

- Why not invite the person you are talking to be sure to interrupt – or otherwise indicate immediately – if anything you say is not clear? And make it crystal clear when switching to a different subject that you are now starting to discuss something new and different. And sum up the main points at the end.

- Watch for the glazed look that shows that the person you are speaking to is no longer listening properly, perhaps because they are still trying to take in the last thing you said.

If necessary, check!

Don't forget that large group of people who politely say they have heard and understood when, in fact, they haven't. One useful way of checking up is to ask in a quiet, friendly way:

'Would you do something for me? Before we go any further, could you tell me what you will say if a friend asks you what I have told you?'

This is not a question to ask every time. But doctors and nurses who never check up in this way – who think only of what a person 'has a right to know' or merely make a note of what they 'have been told' – may remain seriously unaware of the limitations and dangers of communication. Quite commonly, when this question is asked, at least one serious misconception immediately comes to light.

Note that I have here phrased the question in a general way, but it's equally useful in relationship to a particular piece of information:

1   For example, after describing possible side-effects: *'If a friend asks you what side-effects there may be after this treatment that your husband is having, what will you say?'*

2   And after the relative's answer to this question, add another: *'And if you are asked how likely or unlikely it is that each of these side-effects will occur, what will you say?'*

- Watch the face of the person you are talking to (another reason for looking at notes as little as possible). How much is being understood and retained?

- Don't talk too fast or you will not be understood. Nor too slowly or you may be thought patronizing. Vary your speed. Far better than talking slowly and deliberately all the time is to talk in a quick, friendly, almost casual way for part of the time; then slow up for those points that are either so vital that they must be emphasized – or are not at all straightforward and therefore easily missed or misunderstood.

- Repeat some words and phrases, but probably not whole sentences until the end of the interview. There is then less risk of sounding patronizing. Watching a person's face is a big help to knowing what to stress, what to repeat and when to stop and arrange a second interview (which can sometimes be done in a very satisfactory way over the telephone, as discussed later).

- Don't necessarily say everything you originally planned to say. Not now, anyway.

- Sometimes arranging a second interview can actually *save time* in the long run. And never forget that what matters is the actual effect your words are having on the person you are talking to, not the effect you think they ought to have if the relative you are talking to is listening properly.

- Two things are almost certainly going to lead to contradiction and confusion. One is if a relative keeps asking for more and more detail. The other is when a relative keeps asking the same question to different members of staff and comparing what they say. As well as being greedy with staff time (which is not fair to patients and other relatives) many medical situations are quite complex – making contradictions (apparent or real) inevitable when this is done.

To sum up – reminders and options

- Relatives have several roles. They receive information. They provide information. And whether considered as carers or as victims, they may need help.

- Many aspects of good communication can be learned from watching others, from discussions, from going on courses and from workshops.

- You learn all the time, especially from your mistakes. Everyone needs as much feedback as possible as to the actual effect of what they said.

- As with patients, giving information to relatives should always be blended with being *friendly;* with remaining *professional* about what can be done to help, however black the outlook; and with showing at least some *interest* in the patient and relative as people with interesting lives and stories to tell.

- It may be best to give short-term hopes and plans *before* describing what has been found – and how serious it is.

- The way to handle priorities when under pressure is a) to recognize when – because of shock or because saturation point has been reached – to say any more would waste precious time, and b) to give prolonged listening and counselling only to those for whom a brief interview has clearly not been enough.

- Communication must be *realistic*. A very useful question – strongly rec-ommended during or after giving a prognosis or a warning of side-effects, provided it's asked in a gentle, friendly way – is this: 'May I ask you something? How will you reply if a friend asks you what I've said?' The answer can be surprising. Nothing teaches better the art of realistic communication.

References

1   Maguire P (1990) Can Communication Skills Be Taught? *British Journal of Hospital Medicine.* **43**: 215–16.

2   Korsch B M, Freeman B and Negrete V F (1971) Practical Implications of Doctor–Patient Interaction: Analysis for Paediatric Practice. *American Journal of Diseases of Children.* **121**: 110–14.

2

More communication skills and suggestions

Leadership

... by his dignity and his calm self-control in the face of unexpected difficulties he [the physician] checks the excitement of anxious relatives and friends.

(Hippocrates)

Good communication, especially when the relative is demoralized, depressed or frightened, should sometimes have a strong element of *leadership* in it. The qualities needed are very similar to those needed by a good leader in a non-medical emergency or crisis. Qualities such as *staying calm, showing confidence* and *being decisive* may all need to be clearly communicated to an anxious relative. Perhaps not in exactly the same way as to the patient, but in a very similar way.

Strong leadership, or at least the open mention of it, is rather out of fashion at the moment. Sometimes there is a reluctance – even a refusal – to lead. The idea is that patients (and to a greater or less extent relatives) must just be given the facts and then weigh up the pros and cons for themselves. This may sometimes be right, but in practice the perceived ethical and legal advantages are often outweighed by serious disadvantages.

Many patients and relatives are ambivalent. Sometimes they like humility, a doctor who honestly says that he doesn't know. But at other times, often depending on how frightening or serious the situation, these same people – whether patients or relatives – may desperately need from a doctor or nurse the qualities of a good leader, with a measure of confidence and sureness about what needs to be done. After all, to make the point again, in any crisis this is what we all need from a partner or friend. Someone who is not just sympathetic, but who is firm and decisive and who gives us strength.

Experience helps. To have dealt with similar situations gives confidence. But the truth is that doctors *always* have to try and act calmly and confidently. Though their real feelings may be strongly tinged with bewilderment and doubt, all men and women acting as leaders (or as those who have to make quick, firm decisions, whether or not you choose to call it leadership) have to try not to show this.

One kind of leadership is to be very firm, saying little, yet giving confidence – the 'strong and silent' approach. This is something that some health workers carry off very successfully, but which others can't quite get away with. They don't have the personality for it. For them a different approach may be needed, including – whenever there is time for it – explanation and justification at every stage.

Staff nurse to doctor *(after discussing Margaret a four-year-old with an inoperable brain tumour to be treated by radiotherapy)*: *Would you like to hear what Margaret's mother said after you had spent all that time explaining the situation to her? I asked her what you had told her and she replied, 'To tell you the truth, I couldn't tell you a single word he said, but I've complete confidence.'*

Lessons to be learned from this:

- It should have been suspected that this anxious young mother was not taking in what was being said to her. A proper check should then have been made:

  'Before we go any further, may I ask you something? If a friend were to ask you what I have told you so far, *what would you say?'*

- As soon as it became clear that little or nothing was being taken in, a realistic aim would have been to attempt to establish just two key points – not more. And in a gentle, friendly way. Margaret's mother should then have been invited to repeat them – 'to make sure there has been no misunderstanding'.

- Assuming that this could have been done in a few minutes – *and if the same degree of trust* (which can often be judged from the patient's expression) *could also have been achieved during this much shorter time* – it follows that most of the 15 minutes spent on this interview were wasted. These ten minutes could have been spent helping someone else, patient or relative, perhaps someone waiting anxiously to be seen.

- If there is ever a Relative's Charter, it should perhaps say that every relative has a right not to be kept waiting while other relatives are being given detailed information that they are not taking in – or can't handle.

Being positive

Being positive and avoiding being negative are not the same thing, but both are important. A slavish policy of never saying anything in a negative way would be absurd. But in general, if a message can be given in a positive way this will be:

- better understood

- better for morale.

Negative statements can be confusing, especially to those who are anxious and elderly. The message may fail to get across, partly because of its *lack of clarity* and partly because of its *lack of impact.*

Here are some examples of positive statements that may be appropriate:

- 'Good news. Your wife's scan is normal.'

  This is usually better than 'is negative' or 'shows no abnormality'.

- 'This symptom that your mother has started to get is unpleasant for her – and worrying for us. We've been concerned before about such patients, but at least some of them have done well in the end, so let's hope it will be the same with your mother.'

  Negative phrases like 'not necessarily a bad sign' are readily understood by some relatives, but with others may leave an impression that is gloomier than it need be.

- 'Your husband's condition remains serious, but his progress so far is everything we could have hoped for.'

  This could be in reply to 'Is my husband doing as well as you expected?' – a question often asked and one that is surely designed by the relative to make it as easy as possible for the doctor to say something at least a little positive and encouraging.

Being positive overlaps with being optimistic (discussed in Chapters 4 and 5) and with using the powerful psychological weapon of 'suggestion'. Properly used, 'suggestion' can be very valuable and is probably not used enough in mainstream medicine. Used too much, or carried too far, it has the unattractive flavour of high-pressure salesmanship – even of quackery and deception. But it can be of great help, especially during rehabilitation, or when trying to reach goals of any kind. Provided it isn't overdone it can improve quality of life – with only a small risk that it will be later regretted.

Efficiency

To communicate firm, decisive leadership is needed only occasionally – and in fairly critical situations – but to communicate *efficiency* is needed all the time. It's needed to make patients and relatives feel *safe*. It's part of being professional. Relatives know that nobody is perfect and that things can go wrong, but they need to feel that with this doctor, or this nurse, or this team, mistakes are unlikely to occur and that everything will generally run smoothly, with everyone on the same wavelength.

Compared with today, brisk efficiency – and the sheer speed at which they did their work – was what many patients and their relatives admired most in nurses. Perhaps even more than gentleness and kindness, though they certainly liked that too. In those days any chat or counselling had to be very brief and was not expected to the extent it is today.

Consider just four aspects of this vital need for the relative to get a firm impression of efficiency.

- In a situation where *treatment is being varied to suit individual patients,* even though at first sight they have the same problem. Such variation naturally appeals to many patients and relatives because of the attraction of individually tailored care. But the more that standard procedures and treatments are modified, the greater the risk of mistakes, and the greater the risk of confusion. Busy staff, unaware of individual modifications, may tell relatives things about procedures, number of visits, side-effects, etc. that apply to the standard treatment. In an ideal world it wouldn't happen, but it would be foolish not to be realistic about the problem that this poses.

- Both for displaying efficiency and for showing friendly professional interest (see Chapter 1) *a good memory is a priceless asset.* When the doctor's memory is not so good, some relatives will be very understanding about it, but others will be hurt and begin to doubt the sincerity of someone who seems so concerned and interested during a patient's illness – and then only a few months later meets the same relative and looks blankly at her, recalling little or nothing.

Useful tip! If a doctor doesn't have a good memory: a) avoid hospital corridors, local supermarkets, etc. as much as possible, or else walk briskly through them looking neither to the right nor to the left; b) when trapped – and not even sure whether this is a patient, a relative, a member of staff or someone met socially – learn to ask with unhesitating friendly warmth questions like, 'Good to see you again, how are things going?' – and with a bit of luck you will soon have a clue that jogs your memory. It's a bit like admiring a baby when you are not sure whether it's a boy or a girl. Choose your words with care until you get a clue.

- A third aspect of efficiency, often somewhat neglected in large multidisciplinary teams is *avoidance of needless duplication*. Several different members of the same team (and perhaps some from other teams) may talk to the same relative, all asking the same questions.

  This is not always a waste of time because each member of staff does it a little differently and though this may confuse relatives, it may also help them. Also each member of staff and each trainee benefits from hearing things at first hand, rather than just second hand. But a) it may be of very low priority when there is other work to be done, b) it may be exhausting or irritating for the relative, and c) unless the need for it is carefully explained, it may give the relative the impression of an inefficient team, the left hand not knowing what the right hand is doing.

- Finally, efficiency includes *good communication* between different professionals in different departments or different places of work. Relatives will have greater confidence if this is seen to be good. In an ideal world the hospital doctor(s), the family doctor(s), hospital nurses, primary care nurses, social workers and everyone else involved in a difficult case would all be in close touch, following all the subtleties of a changing situation and how patient and relatives are reacting to it.

Sadly in practice it is seldom possible to achieve anywhere near this ideal, either in documentation or in conversation, except for the bare bones of a situation. But whenever it has been possible for different professionals to speak to each other – for example for the hospital doctor to speak to the family doctor – be sure to tell the relative that you have been in touch and made contact with the other doctor. This builds confidence, giving a picture of efficiency rather than muddle.

Who is in the driver's seat?

I have also always felt that in hospital, whenever more than one consultant is involved, it is best for them to agree on which of them shall be regarded, at any one time, as being so to speak, 'in the driver's seat'. Family doctor, patient and relative *must all know who this is.*

Many specialists doubt the need for this. And they are probably not comfortable with any impression that one specialist is senior to another or more concerned than another. But, however closely involved the family doctor, when none of the hospital doctors feels any special responsibility and concern, other than that relating to their own special knowledge and expertise, patient and relatives may fall between two stools and become needlessly demoralized. This is further discussed in Chapter 6.

Rapport and trust

How long should an interview last? Some would say that it can cease when the relative has all the necessary information. But ideally, it should also not end until rapport has been established. *This may sometimes be at least as important as the information given.* If trust can be established with the relative, this can make a big difference to whether or not the *patient* feels the same way, and can also save much precious time in the future.

Sometimes after talking to a relative we can see that the interview has gone well. For example, it's clearly a good sign, if, after hearing what the doctor has to say, a relative initiates a warm handshake and indicates understanding and trust by a friendly offer not to take up any more of the doctor's or nurse's time. Then the interview has achieved one of its most important purposes. But sadly sometimes – in spite of the fact that it is clear that doubts or distrust persist and that we have failed to achieve the sort of rapport we had hoped for – no more time can be spared, at least not at the moment. We should always lean towards blaming ourselves rather than the relative we have been speaking to for this failure, but (as discussed in Chapter 12) the fear and guilt of some relatives may make them distrustful, even hostile, in a way that is very difficult to handle.

Sometimes rapport is quickly achieved with *one* of the relatives of a patient but slowly, if at all, with another. I have a note of how I once spent 25 minutes, which I could ill afford because others were waiting to be seen, talking to the son and daughter of a woman with a brain tumour. If it had been just the daughter, five minutes would have been enough. She made it quite clear that that was all she wanted or needed. But the son remained suspicious and hostile. It was probably right to go on trying to get his trust and understanding. But with hindsight the extra 20 minutes, just for his sake, were wasted.

Unspoken communication

The power of touch

'Now touch the patient' – from instructor to student, as if it must never be omitted – made me cringe the first time I heard it. It's the same with relatives. I have had a warm and close relationship with some relatives, extending over many months of crisis and tragedy, without ever touching them, except perhaps in the most perfunctory way. With this minority it seemed better not to. I am fairly sure that they preferred it that way. You can usually tell.

One man's wife told me that she didn't like it at all when a male nurse, who came to tell her that her husband had died, put his arm around her. It was kindly meant, but for her, at that moment, it was wrong. If you misjudge relatives in this way and they freeze when you touch them, don't take offence or apologize, but quickly take your arm away. On the other hand if they touch you first, respond in the same way immediately, otherwise they may feel that they shouldn't have done it.

There are some distressed relatives who respond to touch by gripping your hand so tightly that it is as if they were drowning and don't ever want to let go. Or perhaps the other hand joins the first and both hands grip yours. You don't need to wonder then if it was the right thing to do. You know it was. And that it was badly needed. And note that this has little or nothing to do with the age or gender of either doctor or relative.

Needless to say those with impaired sight are usually in special need of the comfort and strength that can flow from the right kind of firm, warm touch. I say warm because this is such a help that I have sometimes thought that having warm hands should help to gain entry to medical school.

The right kind of smile

The first thing to be said about smiling is that it is often not remotely connected with humour (*see* quotations in box on the following page). I suppose we could call this 'serious smiling', as opposed to 'humorous smiling', yet somehow that doesn't sound quite right.

'His wise, rare, smile is sweet with certainties'

(from *The Chief,* a sonnet about the surgeon, Lister, by William Henley)

'It was one of those rare smiles with a quality of eternal reassurance in it ... it believed in you as you would like to believe in yourself'

(from *The Great Gatsby* by Scott Fitzgerald)

'But the smile must be of the right kind; and the right kind must have understanding in it, and friendliness, and a good deal of patience'

(from *The Golden Bubble* by Roderic Owen)

Note how these three passages give a fascinating number of ways in which a smile can provide valuable moral support and send all kinds of important messages – messages which have *nothing to do with humour.*

Here are several important messages, quite unconnected with humour, that a warm smile can convey.

- For some relatives the doctor's smile will suggest *understanding* ('I know how you feel')

- For others – *affection* (perhaps too strong a word for the first meeting, but it can be true of subsequent meetings)

- For others – *hope* ('maybe the position is not quite so desperate after all')

- For others – *encouragement* (always a powerful boost to morale)

- For others – *confidence* (the sort of two-way confidence in each other that in the non-medical world, just as much as in the medical world, cements relationships).

If there's one thing that can never be taught, or copied, or practised, it's this kind of warm smile, unconnected with humour. It doesn't need to be a big smile. It may be very slight, yet unmistakable – partly because a warm smile is always reflected in the eyes as well as in the lips. If it's a natural part of your personality then – whether doctor or nurse, male or female – it can be a great asset.

As with every other aspect of this fragile, subtle, impossible-to-describe world of unspoken communication, *there's a right time to smile and a wrong time to smile.* And it must come from the heart. A relative may perhaps occasionally be fooled into thinking that a warm smile is genuine when it isn't, but not often. Patients and their relatives can usually tell.

Perhaps the most remarkable thing of all is the ability of a smile to give patients or relatives more confidence, not just in the doctor or nurse, but *in themselves.* How do you explain that? I have no idea. Strange, but true.

Humour

The health worker who can't manage the occasional use of the right kind of humour is also missing out on a valuable weapon in the fight against low morale. Not what Anthony Trollope called 'the oppressive cheerfulness of some doctors', but sincere good humour of the kind exchanged between friends. I once knew a doctor who always had a new story to make his friends and colleagues smile, but it seemed that not one of the patients or relatives he spoke to ever heard any of them. He was kind enough, but his ward rounds were like funeral processions. How sad.

It's true that humour in a serious situation can be a disaster if it misfires, yet that should be rare – it's too valuable to omit for that reason. Fear grows less and tension is eased. As with leadership, it's not just a medical matter. For many people humour can sharply reduce stress and fear in *any* kind of crisis. In the middle of a night battle in the North African desert in 1942, the sand littered with burning tanks and exploding ammunition and everyone faced with the possibility that at any moment they could be blown to pieces, a voice was suddenly heard to say quietly, 'I still say it's not as good as Blackpool illuminations' – and everyone felt better and less afraid.

There is a remarkable ambivalence about humour in the presence of serious illness. If anything light-hearted that a doctor has written in a patient's case notes is read out in Court, it can be used to make the doctor sound like a monster. Yet in real life it can dramatically reduce stress for both patients, relatives and staff – without anyone finding it in bad taste.

It certainly need not suggest any lack of concern. Quite the reverse. Don't forget that it's quite common in dramas for the doctor with the best sense of humour to be also the most caring. This was well shown in M.A.S.H., the American television series about a medical unit in the Korean war. The wise-cracking doctors with their black humour were also the most understanding and the most caring. The ones with little or no sense of humour tended to be less caring and less effective.

Humour is a matter of personal taste and can easily go cold and sound embarrassingly unfunny when any attempt is made to reproduce it in print. Nevertheless many doctors and nurses find that it can help relatives to cope with their fear – for example, when a patient is first admitted to hospital.

FIRST EXAMPLE

Doctor *(with mock seriousness, to tall, dark-haired patient from Wales in the presence of her husband)*: *One final thing I want to tell you both – recent research suggests that this treatment works best with tall, dark-haired women living in Wales.*

Nurse *(a few minutes later to second nurse after they have both overheard this)*: *He's full of blarney, isn't he?*

Second nurse: *Maybe. But then she hasn't heard it before, like you and I have. And you must admit, he's quite good at picking the right patient for it. You can see it was right for her, she liked it; she's looking more relaxed and less scared already. Not like Doctor X who tries the same joke with every patient and then wonders why some miss the point and are not helped in the least.*

SECOND EXAMPLE

Doctor *(to very nervous, newly admitted patient and relative, with nurse present and in a ward where the immediate impression is that the regime is very friendly and relaxed)*: *I must first warn you that the nurses in this ward are very strict.*

THIRD EXAMPLE

Doctor *(seeing 80-year-old patient and relative both looking very tense)*: *You are 80, aren't you? Well, the good news is that this week we are offering anyone over your age a free 80 000 mile check-up …*

Humour and compassion make good companions. Even mock bullying, or mock lack of sympathy, or talk of strict discipline. Be careful, but some patients and some relatives feel a lot better for it. Humorous cartoons on a notice board for patients and relatives to see – usually about the funny side of life in hospital – are nearly always popular and help to take away fear. And, of course, when you know a patient or relative you get to know their kind of humour.

The telephone

As a means of communicating with relatives the telephone is probably not used enough.

• It can be very useful for a second interview, adding points that were not made in the first interview because it was felt that saturation point had been reached.

• It may also provide, not so much information, as powerful moral support, usually following a previous face-to-face interview, but sometimes even when the relative has never met the doctor or nurse concerned.

Given the importance in normal conversation of various forms of unspoken communication, it's surprising how effective the telephone can be. I've never ceased to be surprised by this and don't fully understand it (but don't forget how warm and personal it can be in the case of lovers – neither can see the other, but there's nothing impersonal about it – it can be pure magic).

One thing I found very useful in my later years as a hospital consultant – and wished I'd done sooner – was to ask the nursing staff to wait until the patient's partner paid his evening visit, and then to 'phone my home and see if I was in. If I was (and if I was thoroughly conversant with the patient's situation, so not needing the hospital case notes – and wasn't in the middle of entertaining friends), the nurse would tell the relative that I was on the 'phone from my home and ask her if she'd like to have a word with me. Or alternatively tell her that I'd appreciate having a word with her to get her opinion or advice.

This can be very useful for the busy hospital doctor, perhaps preparing a lecture at home or trying to write an article. One of the reasons for this, I think, is that there is something friendly and caring about the doctor speaking from his own home, when off duty, which may fully compensate for not staying late at the hospital in order to talk face-to-face. But, as with so much else suggested in this book, some relatives may like it, some may not; and it may suit some doctors but not others.

Impaired hearing

- Especially with elderly relatives, remember the possibility that their hearing may be impaired – and that they will be reluctant to admit to this.

- Never forget something equally important – that there may be nothing wrong with their hearing, but they can't take things in as quickly as they used to. Just because they don't immediately catch the gist of what you say doesn't mean that you necessarily need to speak any louder.

    Ideally, information on these two points would come to hospital staff from GPs but, for various reasons, it seldom does – just as GPs frequently don't get from hospitals the sort of practical information they need if they are to 'treat the patient and not just the disease'.

- When impairment is suspected (or seems quite likely just from age) the most tactful thing may be not to discuss the matter, but just to *shut all doors and windows* (which not only helps privacy but also cuts out other sounds) and then follow a few simple suggestions, which – unlike talking loudly – will not give offence should hearing in fact be quite good.

- Look for a hearing aid inserted in either ear, and whenever you see one, don't forget that hearing is unlikely to be restored completely to normal. It may still be quite impaired or distorted.

- Unless you really *have* to, don't talk especially loudly or slowly, because it is almost impossible to do so without sounding disrespectful (quite apart from the loss of confidentiality).

- Don't forget that lip reading may be *wholly or partly* relied on by the person you are speaking to. Face him (an important exception to the advice given in Chapter 1 about adopting a less formal position) and talk normally and naturally. Make sure that your face is in a good light. Never talk while looking down or turning your head away.

- Sometimes before leaving ask, 'Is there any point I've mentioned that you would like me to write down – to remind you what I have said?' ('to remind you' is more tactful than 'in case there is anything you haven't heard clearly or understood properly').

A few key points

- When there are difficult decisions to be made, relatives may sometimes appreciate a doctor who merely gives facts and options, but at other times they might regard such lack of leadership and support as unhelpful.

- Whenever possible express things in a positive rather than a negative way, and also have a positive attitude to what can be done.

- Even with the worst possible prognosis, efficiency and avoidance of muddle or duplication of effort may be as important as kindness. Special care is needed when standard treatments are tailored to suit individual needs.

- When two or more senior hospital staff in different specialties are involved, as quite often happens, it is best for them to agree on which of them at any one time is to be 'in the driver's seat'. Being in this position means not just offering special expertise, but also feeling responsible for the overall picture from the hospital angle and being the consultant mainly responsible for communicating with enquiring relatives. Patient, relatives and GP should all know who this is.

- Occasional humour – of the right kind, at the right time – can be an antidote to gloom and fear and a boost to the morale of anxious relatives. But if it does not suit a doctor's personality – if feedback shows that for him or her it is misfiring or not helping patients or relatives in the way hoped – it may be something to leave to others.

- Talking to relatives on the 'phone is not as impersonal as it sounds; it can be very valuable. But, as with everything, it works better with some doctors (and perhaps with some relatives) than with others.

- Remember the possibility that relatives either have impaired hearing or an impaired ability to take in immediately what is said to them. Several simple measures, too often neglected, may avoid any need to speak louder than normal.

3

Who? When? Where?

Do we wait for relatives to request an interview? Or do we routinely ask for one? Most relatives are very considerate and reasonable, but:

- some feel that they should not have to ask, but should be automatically invited

- others may object to being asked when they have not requested it.

All this may be tied up with emotional ambivalence, anger and guilt, especially when the relative is the son or daughter of an elderly patient who lives alone.

It is also not so uncommon for relatives to prefer *not* to see a doctor if they think that all they get will be bad news, destroying all hope. And some, though they might not admit it, are not really sure whether or not they want information of any kind. Then 'floating anger' (*see* Chapter 12) may cause them to complain later that they were not fully informed, when this was at least partly of their own choosing. So staff sometimes have a feeling that they can't win. But no doctor or nurse must mind if criticized first for one thing, then for the opposite.

If requested to attend for interview, some relatives become alarmed, fearing that this may mean very bad news. To avoid this, it may be best for whoever arranges the interview:

- to stress that, in this unit, to see the relatives is a routine matter (or perhaps 'Doctor X likes to see all relatives')

- to stress that in this case the medical staff would like to *exchange* information and to hear the relative's views (or perhaps 'Doctor Y would like to meet you and have a chat – he'd like to know what you think').

Most of the public – and most nursing staff – feel that, in general, it's best that serious bad news should come from medical, rather than nursing, staff.

And some feel that it is wrong to have junior doctors do it. Perhaps senior staff should give the matter more priority. But the reality is that, in many units, for senior staff to take responsibility for this as a routine would mean that they would either have to do it very briefly or else accept serious inroads into their other work.

Some relatives (but not as many as there used to be) will be happy just to assume that the doctor or the team will do their best – and that staff are far too busy to be explaining everything to everyone. Others will want a considerable amount of information before trust and rapport is achieved.

It's often – but not always – best to ask the patient before seeing the relative. Those critics who think that we should *always* do this (unless the patient is too ill or too confused to give permission) may be correct in a strict legal sense (*see* box in Chapter 1) but are usually imagining themselves to be not a relative, but a patient – and thinking of it purely from this point of view.

They may feel differently if they imagine themselves to be a relative, desperately anxious about a sick or injured loved one. They might not be very happy if a doctor or nurse were to say, 'I'm sorry, I can say nothing until your mother gives formal permission'. Common sense is needed, not just slogans.

Should patient and relative be seen together? The two extremes here are the old idea of *never* seeing the patient and relative together, and the new one in which some doctors are said to be reluctant to talk to a relative *except* with the patient present. Most doctors and nurses don't fall into either extreme. They vary what they do according to the situation and their assessment of each person involved.

Examples of what a doctor might say in various different circumstances when a relative is visiting a patient in hospital:

- **Doctor to patient (*his wife at bedside*)**: *May I now have a few words with your wife alone? I want to hear her impression of how you have been lately. And I want to explain things to her and answer any questions she may have. We'll come back soon. Then the three of us can have a chat.*

- **Doctor to patient (*his wife waiting outside*)**: *Now, for the rest of what I want to say, how about having your wife join us? That way you will be able to remind each other of what the tests show and what you and I have decided is the next step that needs to be taken.*

There is one thing that I have often done since early in my career and feel is valuable and important – to try and persuade relatives that, at the end of an interview at which the patient is not present, *doctor and relative immediately go together to the patient.* Many relatives are at first reluctant to do this, especially if the outlook is very bad, but later, in my experience, are usually glad they did so. Fear and tension are reduced. And it's good for the patient's dignity and self-respect that doctor and relative should appear together like this – quite openly in a natural, unafraid way – willing to discuss anything the patient wants to discuss.

It can also help the relative to hear how the doctor talks to the patient:

- not saying anything untrue, yet giving maximum encouragement and boosting morale in various ways, especially being as positive as possible about the immediate future

- talking in a natural, relaxed way, with a brief but friendly 'irrelevant' question or comment about the past life of the patient or relative

- showing a sincere interest in every symptom and every problem, together with an obvious desire to do something about each one, regardless of how bad the prognosis.

Surprisingly, at such a meeting, it may be that there is no discussion of either diagnosis or prognosis. That doesn't matter. It can come later. There are always other things to talk about, especially plans for the immediate future. Moreover experience shows that this is one of those occasions when, provided there is a good trusting doctor–patient and doctor–relative relationship, a sense of humour about the less serious aspects of the situation may be of surprising help to all concerned. Humour of the right kind (with no deception) is shared by all three – patient, relative and doctor – and sometimes the worst of the cold fear and sadness suddenly melts like snow in warm sunshine.

But beware! Unless able to display effortless friendly professional interest, in spite of having just given bad news, it may be better *not* to go back to the patient with the relative in this way. If the doctor or nurse is going to look sad, awkward, cold or embarrassed, the exercise will founder and may do more harm than good.

Large families

Large families, with a strong family feeling, are not nearly so common as they used to be. But occasionally, when there are several anxious relatives

– for example when the oldest surviving member of a large family may not have long to live – it may be best to arrange a special meeting, either in hospital or in the patient's home, and speak to several at the same time. Perhaps one or more sons or daughters flies in from America or some other part of the world, and it may then be especially important to explain everything to them and convince them that everything that is right and possible is being done.

This idea of an interview with several relatives together may be resisted by one or more of them, either because the person nearest to the patient objects to sharing interviews with more distant relatives, or because of friction in the family. For example, there can be bad feeling between those relatives who had the burden of caring for the patient and others who drop in near the end, having previously not offered any help. And sometimes one relative will be keen to give an opinion or to pass on to the doctor some information about the patient (reliable or otherwise) that he doesn't want others in the family to hear.

Occasionally things get quite complicated because the patient has been leading a double life, perhaps romantically involved with two people, neither of them aware of the existence of the other.

But in general, if it can be arranged, such an interview:

- helps to save time – no need to keep repeating the same things to different members of the family

- helps the aim of being even-handed – not causing bad feeling by talking, for example, to one son or daughter but not to another

- helps understanding – those who have listened and understood best can later correct any wrong ideas that others may have about what they heard.

As with a single relative, if it seems that a good rapport has been achieved, why not round off the interview by warmly and sincerely shaking hands with every relative present? It can help to cement a lasting trust.

Appoint a spokesperson?

It is sometimes best with a large family – either from the very start or after an initial interview with several relatives – for the family to agree to one of them being the *key representative* and for all communication to be done in future through this one person. This is especially necessary in the case of a long illness of an elderly patient with many concerned relatives.

Is there a key person in the family? Who is the strongest? Someone that others trust and confide in. This person can be the one that others 'phone. The next of kin is not always the main helper, or carer, or leader in a crisis. Having met several members of the family, doctors and nurses may have their own views on who they hope this spokesperson will be – or not be! Just as there can be 'heartsink' patients, so there can be 'heartsink' relatives. Of course, staff may get it wrong. The most articulate, the most extrovert, the most apparently confident, the sort picked out to speak on television programmes, sometimes turns out to be by no means the strongest or the most sensible.

Finally, it goes without saying that if a patient with no partner has strong views on who should be the spokesperson, that may override anything the family may decide among themselves – or any views the staff may have.

Hospital doctor and family doctor

I shudder to think how often a GP, knowing the family far better than me, has smiled at how wrong my initial assessment of family members has been. In such a case, would it not be better to leave communication with the family to the family doctor? This has obvious advantages – and used to be routinely advised – but is seldom practicable these days for the following reasons.

- Most relatives now feel they have a right to immediate first hand, on-the-spot information – specialized and technical if necessary.

- There are many situations in which they are likely to resent it if the hospital doctor declines to discuss the situation on the grounds that it will be best left to the GP.

- Such delay can cause extreme – perhaps needless – anxiety.

Later, of course, a chance to talk over with their GP what they were told (or think they were told) at the hospital may be very helpful. Knowing the relative better (and perhaps being better at explaining technical matters in plain language) the family doctor may do a vital job of clarification – and of damage limitation should there have been any serious misunderstanding.

There are also many other occasions on which the hospital doctor will advise relatives to go to their family doctor for advice and moral support. For example, when they have had bad news and worry about whether or not to pass it on to a child or an elderly relative – and, if so, how to do it.

So if hospital specialists frequently have to break bad news to relatives, how can they be better briefed on each occasion? Here are four examples of helpful advice passed on to me from family doctors, which I jotted down at the time as being the sort of thing that ought to happen more often.

- 'Be careful when you talk to her husband; I find he is very liable to mis-quote what you tell him.'

- 'You may like to know that her mother died of cancer and had a very bad time'.

- 'If you are seeing his wife, I advise you to try and have the eldest daughter present; she has far more sense than her mother and will help to see that you are not misquoted'.

- 'Her husband was a patient of yours ten years ago.' (Very useful for doctors or nurses whose memory for names and faces is not as good as they would like.)

All are important points that could be of great help to the specialist before he talks to the patient or relative about diagnosis and prognosis.

Unfortunately it has now become even harder to pass on confidential personal information of this kind. More and more people seem especially to disapprove of anything in medical records that sounds 'judgemental'. Doctors are supposed to operate not in the real world, but in a world where all relatives are equally intelligent and reliable. Which, of course, they are not. Any more than are all doctors or all nurses.

Extract from a letter sent by a hospital doctor to a family doctor:

This patient's wife and son have both seemed to me more illogical and unpredictable than is usual in this sort of situation. Sometimes grateful, sometimes critical, sometimes understanding and sometimes talking as if the situation had never been explained to them (though it has been explained several times). No doubt there are underlying emotional reasons for all this.

True, if such helpful information is written down, there is a danger that the patient or relatives may read it and any existing family friction be further exacerbated. Letters given to take to the hospital were always liable to be opened by the relative. Every sensible doctor knew that. But now medical records are available for inspection by any patient or relative – though with certain restrictions.

As regards information flowing from hospital to GP, there are in this case even greater imperfections and defects that frustrate family doctors. Some hospital doctors try harder than others to improve matters, but it's an uphill struggle. Ideally, at the very least the following should be noted.

- If a patient dies in hospital or hospice, a message to this effect (no details needed) should be 'phoned to the GP's surgery *immediately*. It's upsetting for relatives and embarrassing for the GP if they meet a day or two later and the GP has no idea that the patient has died.

- When a patient is discharged home (preferably not at the weekend, unless this is unavoidable) there should be:

  – a 'phone message to say the patient is going home

  – a brief report on the day of discharge

  – a full report not too far behind it.

  Delays before a full report is in the hands of the GP are still far too common. In many hospitals there is delay before a full report is dictated and further delay before it is typed. Some units have tried sending a report out a few days before discharge, but there are obvious problems about this.

Finally, *never accept too literally what a patient or relative claims that another doctor said*. Apart from anything else, this may be very unfair to a colleague. Rather than asking, 'Are you sure he really said that?', just say that you would be interested to hear more of exactly what was said. And be sure to ask for both sides of the conversation. To give a fair assessment of what a doctor (or anyone else for that matter) is quoted as saying, you need to know if it was said in reply to a question and, if so, what the question was.

How many professionals?

How many professionals should be present when relatives are interviewed in hospital? Just one is more intimate. But there are distinct advantages – whenever time permits – to having a junior nurse or doctor present when a more senior member of staff conducts an interview. They hear what is said. And if they like what they hear and feel it was well done, they can pick up some useful tips.

My experience is that most relatives don't mind another person being present, so long as:

- the reason is explained to them – everyone understands the need to learn

- just one other person is present – two is too many

- this extra person is unobtrusive and just an observer, not making any comment in front of the relative

- at the end of the interview the student is asked to leave and the doctor has a moment or two alone with the relative, who may have something to say without anyone else being present

- only after this, and the relative has left, does the interviewer discuss with the nurse, doctor or student what was said, how the relative reacted and so on.

Doctor *(concluding an interview with the parents of a 16-year-old girl)*: *Let's go and see her together now.*

Mother: *Do you think we should? Don't you think it would be better not? I don't want her to see me like this.*

Doctor: *I can understand how you feel, but I hope you'll come with me. She knows I'm seeing you. Let's show her that we are not afraid to talk to her.*

Father *(to wife)*: *I agree with the doctor. It won't matter if she sees you looking a bit upset. She'll understand…*

Two senior doctors seeing the relative together

It used to be thought essential, or at least highly desirable, for the GP to be present whenever a specialist saw patients in their own home, and for these two doctors to be together if the GP then invited the specialist to talk to relatives in another room and answer any questions. I used to think so, too. A chance to meet together. Each hears everything that the other says. And in some ways good for the patient to see her two leading doctors together. But I fairly soon came to prefer to see the patient alone; and then go straight to see the GP alone at his or her surgery to talk over the situation. This is because, when more than one doctor is present the doctor–patient, or doctor–relative, relationship always seems to suffer. I don't know quite why, but it does. Hugh Barber agreed: 'It is not always easy', he wrote, 'for a doctor to leave a house more contented for his visit... when there are two doctors it may be twice as difficult.'[1]

The same thing applies when two hospital doctors see patients or relatives together at a joint clinic. In many ways it is an excellent idea. Each learns from the other. They discuss what seems best for each patient. Experience is pooled. In the treatment of cancer, for example, one may be trained to carry out surgery, the other radiotherapy or chemotherapy. But something of importance is lost. It seems that there can't be the same warm relationship when two doctors try to share it. As for more than two it was Sir William Osler who wrote that there surely cannot be anything 'more doleful' than four or five doctors entering a patient's room together.

Similarly if a senior doctor and a senior nurse are going to share breaking bad news to a relative (a combination that can in my experience be very useful), it might seem important that they stay together so that each can hear what the other says – or at least for the one who goes second to have been present from the start and so know what has been said.

However:

- two staff, instead of one, become unavailable for other work. Many units are just too busy to adopt this practice as a routine

- as mentioned above, something is lost. The patient will be helped more if seen by sympathetic staff *separately*, not together

- when a doctor and nurse work well together as a team, they don't usually need to know what the other has already said. *Better to ask the relative*, then deal with any obvious misconceptions or vital point missed. In either case, *what the relative has retained* from the interview is what matters, not what the first speaker actually said or didn't say.

When giving bad news is shared in this way, it doesn't seem to matter who goes first, doctor or nurse, provided the first to go explains who will be following them.

Useful reminders and options

- When asking relatives to attend for interview it may be best in order to limit anxiety either to explain that with this unit, or this doctor, this is a routine matter – or to stress that the view of the relative will help the doctors.

- Whether in hospital or in the patient's home it's often a good idea, at the end of an interview away from the patient, for doctor and relative to go to the patient together and for the three to talk together for a bit (not necessarily about diagnosis or prognosis) before the doctor leaves. Initial reluctance is common, but in most cases relatives are later glad that they were persuaded to do this.

- Sometimes it may be best to see several relatives together, and then, if necessary, to agree on just one who will pass on news to the others.

- In hospital practice relatives may greatly value a talk with the family doctor in due course but these days are seldom prepared to wait for this before learning how serious things are. They want to hear first hand what the hospital doctor has to say.

- Under certain strict conditions it usually seems permissible, in the interest of training, for just one student or junior doctor to be present as an observer when bad news is being given to a relative.

- At first sight it sounds like a good idea for two professionals (specialist and GP, or two specialists, or nurse and doctor) to talk to a relative together, so that each hears what the other one says. But the relationship with the relative seems to suffer too much for this to be recommended as a general policy. It lacks the warmth and empathy of a good consultation with just one person.

Reference

1   Barber H (1947) *The Occasion Fleeting*. H K Lewis, London.

Diagnosis and prognosis

This book is concerned only with serious situations. But how serious is serious? It is neither necessary nor possible to attempt an exact definition, but I suppose that serious means to most people a situation that poses a major threat – in the short term or in the longer term – either to survival or to a reasonable quality of life.

These days, more than ever before, relatives may hear the diagnosis from the patient before they hear it from the doctor. Or perhaps patient and relative are told together. But that doesn't mean that when relatives see the doctor alone they will not have questions to ask. There is still today much less bluntness about prognosis than there is about diagnosis. So relatives may well wonder whether there was anything important that it was thought better not to spell out to the patient, who, don't forget, may be weak, ill, elderly, depressed or excessively fearful.

When the diagnosis is in doubt

Sometimes doctors have to discuss diagnosis and prognosis with relatives before all the tests are complete, or at a clinical stage when nothing definite can yet be said. They would be failing in their job if they did not frequently consider the *possibility* of something serious. It used to be thought foolish and thoughtless to pass this possibility straight on to an anxious patient or relative, but now there is increasing pressure on doctors to do so, to say to a relative, for example, 'I have to tell you that it is *possible* that your wife may turn out to have multiple sclerosis'.

If this is done it may be best to advise relatives to keep it to themselves, as it is unlikely that the word 'possible' will be retained for long, even if correctly understood and accurately quoted by the relative who heard it first. It spoils the dramatic effect. What is no more than a possibility soon becomes regarded, as it is passed from one person to another, as a probability or even a certainty. Truth is rapidly turned into untruth. When the risk of the story being changed in this way is stressed some relatives will heed the advice not to pass it on, but many will be unable to resist the temptation.

A similar problem arises when the result of a cervical smear test for cancer is not quite normal. For many women and their relatives the psychological impact when told of any doubt is devastating. Many patients and relatives will go through a period of great anguish and anxiety that may well turn out to have been needless. Nevertheless at the moment this approach rather than traditional restraint, seems to be what society wants.

Needless or exaggerated fears on hearing the diagnosis

When the diagnosis is certain, should we ask relatives how much they know about the condition? Since we don't want to seem to be testing their knowledge in a way that could make them feel foolish, a better way is to ask them if they have ever *known anyone suffering from it*. This is a very useful question and the answer should be *recorded* for other staff to see. The reply (for example, 'Yes, and she had a terrible time and finished paralysed' or 'No, but I have always understood that it's soon fatal') will often bring to light various misconceptions or exaggerated fears needing correction. For example, if leukaemia is the diagnosis, it may allow the relative to be assured that there are several types and that what happened to the person they know – or heard about, or read about – may be irrelevant. It may have been a different kind of leukaemia with a different prognosis.

So exaggerated are the fears of certain diagnostic labels, for example cancer, that a euphemism may sometimes give a more correct and truthful impression than does a curt statement. But the present swing towards giving blunt diagnostic labels makes it harder to be flexible and to treat each person as an individual.

There is a danger of paying lip service to truth telling without paying too much attention to the truthfulness of the impression created. The young doctor may sleep well because he has 'told the truth', but the patient may lie awake with exaggerated fears. It's important to be realistic and to recognize that lifelong misconceptions about a diagnostic label may be quite impervious to a single interview that attempts to correct them.

Cancer is probably the chief problem, but the same thing applies to many other conditions. The true situation is often bad enough without needless fears. When there is no reason to think that either infection or heredity play a part, for example, there is an especial need to make this quite clear.

A single statement may not be adequate. You may have to convince people in more ways than one, according to your assessment of the person you are speaking to and the feedback you get from them as you attempt to reassure them.

Doctor X: *I'm afraid your wife's problem is serious, but I want to say...*

Distressed relative (interrupting): *You mean there's no hope?*

Doctor X (with sincere warmth and feeling): *Oh no, you mustn't think that. It's not that bad. It's certainly serious, but I can assure you it's not hopeless. We've had patients as bad as your wife who have done well. She still has a chance.*

(This relative then – rather unwisely – decides to ask to see another doctor on the team, without revealing that he has already seen Doctor X.)

Relative to Doctor Y: *Do you agree that there is at least some hope for my wife?*

Doctor Y (looking embarrassed and awkward): *Well, I suppose you could say it's not completely hopeless, but... er... well... I'm afraid it does look extremely bad.*

(Relative now not only plunged back into despair, but feels confused and bitter that the two doctors should give what seem to him different opinions.)

But note that, in fact, Doctor X and Doctor Y:

- don't disagree about the prognosis – they agree

- are both being equally truthful and sincere, but the *effect* of their words is quite different because of the way they have said them, the different emphasis and the different manner (one warm, the other cold).

The relative is now thoroughly depressed again. Those who don't believe in any optimism when the outlook is serious may feel that this is unavoidable, even desirable. But there was nothing untrue in what the first doctor said. Hasn't the relative's distress been needlessly increased by the second doctor, who has merely made the situation harder for him to bear?

- *Heredity*: One or other side of the family may be wrongly blamed. Or perhaps it is feared that brothers or sisters or children could also develop the condition because it is now 'in the family'.

- *Infection*: There may be needless fear of visiting (especially by children), of touching or of coughing, of sharing eating utensils, or towels or a bed.

- *Punishment*: Cancer is not only regarded by many people as something unnatural, evil and horrible, but it also seems more likely than other conditions to be regarded as a punishment. My impression is that such feelings are much more common than is generally realized.

- *Stigma*: Whenever possible, say 'It could happen to anyone, it could have happened in my family'. Just these few words can be very effective and may render unnecessary any detailed exploration of hidden fears, private problems and so on (embarrassing for the relative and time-consuming for the doctor).

- *Short-term fears*: 'Will we ever have another holiday together?', 'Will he still be alive by Christmas?' Due to the shock of the diagnosis, such fears are often excessively pessimistic.

- *Long-term fears* of various kinds may also be exaggerated.

- *Gloomy fears of inevitable suffering*, sometimes fuelled by media reports, or by fund raising advertisements for medical charities.

Giving bad news

- It may be a good idea to start the interview (as suggested in Chapter 1) with the plan of action for the immediate future, especially the approximate date when it is hoped that a hospital patient will be able to go home.

- Then, turning to diagnosis and prognosis, ask 'To save time, what do you know so far? What have you been told already?'

- Next (*see* Chapter 1) don't be tied by the logical sequence of always giving the diagnosis before the prognosis. It's sometimes better to *reverse the order*, briefly giving the prognosis first, especially if it seems likely that the diagnosis will be such a shock that nothing after that will be remembered.

Then, whether you are talking to a patient or a relative, I suggest there are broadly three ways of giving bad news, the third way usually being the best.

1   The first is the brief and blunt way. Perhaps the doctor who does it this way is just clumsy and thoughtless. But perhaps he or she honestly believes that bad news can never be anything but bad news, that the patient who is very upset may nevertheless appreciate the bluntness (this is sometimes true) and that there is no point in prolonging things.

2   The second way is to be concerned, unhurried, sad and sympathetic, but how the relative is reacting is not allowed to have much effect on the painful duty of delivering the bad news, which is given as planned before the interview began. Also any good news or positive plans tend to be left until all the bad news has been given. The snags about this are that the pain and shock are greater than they need be. And it's very easy for the relative to get the impression that the situation is hopeless when it isn't. 'Very serious' and 'hopeless' are two different things.

3   The third way of giving bad news includes – *from the very start of the interview* – blending positive statements and plans for the immediate future with the bad news. To the person you are talking to this can make a big difference. Without saying anything misleading or untrue the blow is less harsh, less cruel, easier to bear.

Here are three examples of the sort of thing that can be said. None is appropriate in every case, but one or more may be useful when no really effective treatment has yet been discovered.

- 'At least you'll be glad that your husband's tests are all finished and that we now know what the trouble is and what we are up against.'

- 'Statistically it looks bad – he couldn't get life insurance cover – but there are always some in this situation who do far better than average and he could be one.'

- 'You can never be sure when research is going to make a breakthrough, and I can promise you it's going on all the time.'

More examples are given in Chapter 5 when optimism is discussed.
    It's important to stress that what is said in the third way (unlike the two other ways) depends partly on how the person reacts. There should be

constant *feedback* from the relative you are speaking to. Watch the face, especially the eyes. Then you know when to repeat or stress a word or phrase – and when to change direction.

As mentioned in Chapter 1 you also learn to recognize the *glazed look* that tells you that the person you are talking to is no longer listening. This can come on very early in the interview from shock, or not until later when saturation point has been reached. Either way, *this is the time to stop.* Perhaps make one final attempt to get across one brief, simple, yet balanced message – for example, 'Serious, but *not* hopeless' – then *stop* and perhaps arrange a *second interview,* which can sometimes take place in a fairly brief and surprisingly satisfactory way on the telephone, as suggested in Chapter 1.

- Sometimes it helps if the doctor has the confidence to be *silent* while what has been said sinks in. On the other hand if, at the wrong moment, you just sit there saying nothing, the relative you are speaking to may wonder why you have suddenly dried up. It may then seem that, though sympathetic, you lack the strength and confidence that he needs to support him. It's all a question of a 'feel' for the right timing. As Richard Asher put it, the art is knowing 'when to probe and when to leave alone, when to chide and when to reassure, when to speak and when to keep silent'.[1]

- It's sometimes said, don't give the bad news all at once, keep some for later, but you have to be careful about this and do it only in such a way that you don't lose long-term trust.

- Don't forget that some relatives will be anxious not to take up too much of the doctor's time, and that others may actually prefer a fairly brusque and business-like approach. Even when the news is very bad they may prefer a *minimum* of sympathy and sentiment. Yet even here there should be an element of friendship and understanding.

- The second kind of feedback, which is especially valuable in enabling you to learn from your mistakes, is hearing later from others (staff, patient, or other relatives) about the effect of what you said – after the person you were talking to had had time to digest it. The relative may be more optimistic – or more pessimistic – than you intended. Either may need to be corrected. Yet sometimes it seems wiser not to be in too much of a hurry to do so. This is discussed in Chapter 5.

Giving bad news to a relative is not a painful duty to be carried out once and then forgotten.

- However well the initial interview seems to have gone, a further meeting may reveal persistent misunderstandings.

- More detail may be needed. A common mistake is to give too much detail in the first interview, ignoring the fact that a relative in a state of shock can't possibly take it all in – none of us could. However, even in a second interview, detail is *not* always needed.

- The prognosis may change. Following treatment, or even without any treatment, the patient may do unusually well – or unusually badly.

- Quite apart from this, the attitude of the relative can alter, just as can that of the patient, requiring a different kind of support, with a different emphasis.

- A remark by a friend, a letter from another patient, a newspaper headline or a television programme can all cause a sudden change in morale.

Doctor *(to relative after giving bad news)*: *That's it then. I'm sorry I had to give you bad news, but it could happen to anyone, we don't know anything about the cause. Statistically it looks bad, but you never know. Some patients – I wish it were more, but at least it's a few – are alive and well years later. Your wife is no worse than other patients we have had who have done well. There's no reason why she should not be another of the lucky ones. Good-bye then … (shaking hands) … and let me know if you want to see me again.*

Note that the doctor is here stressing certain points that he has already made while giving the bad news.

It's irresponsible to concentrate on saying things that are true without paying much attention to whether or not this leaves a truthful impression. When we are doing our best for individual people – who, after all, are not robots but all different – we have to consider the likely effect *on this particular relative, at this particular time,* of what is said – not what it logically ought to be, nor what it would have been if the same relative had been spoken to in the same way last month, when her mood was different.

'When will we know whether or not he is cured?'

When there is a chance of cure – even a small one – this is a common question, especially for cancer. Somehow the message has to be got across that there can never be any proof that cure has been achieved – no test can say definitely whether a patient is cured or not – but that it is a matter of probabilities, and that these probabilities may be strong or weak and will change with time.

> **How important is it to the relatives that the prognosis is as accurate as possible? Hippocrates (writing nearly 2,500 years ago) thought it of supreme importance. At the other extreme are those doctors who say, 'Don't give a prognosis, it's bound to be wrong.' Or 'You can't give a prognosis in an individual case.' Which seems to me far too negative. There is no more – and no less – certainty in medicine than there is in many other walks of life; but probabilities and possibilities can be important and helpful, provided it is accepted that that is all they are.**

Misquoting the prognosis

When a relative is told several things in the course of a single interview, the danger of misconception and misquoting is bound to be very real, just as it is in any walk of life. After all, if roles are reversed and it is the doctor in his private life asking some non-medical expert for options and the reasons for them – together with various other details – he is very liable to misunderstand and to misquote.

> **Perhaps the doctor should more often make this point to patients and relatives; 'When I have someone explaining something to me', he or she might say to a relative, 'say my plumber or my bank manager, I often get lost unless they take it very slowly and, even then, I'm sure I'm liable to misquote them.' But don't forget that such humility and realism, though greatly appreciated by some relatives, will sound to others weak and lacking in the sort of confidence that they expect a doctor to show.**

When the situation is very emotional, even the briefest message may be misquoted: 'Do you mean my wife might have only a few weeks to live?' asks the relative, and the doctor replies that, yes, that is sadly the *average* sort of time in this situation. Or perhaps the average is quite a lot better than that, but the doctor says that she *might* have only six months to live because he believes it best for the family to be prepared for this serious *possibility*. Then neighbours pass around the word that 'The doctor says she has only six months to live'. And every month beyond this is regarded as proof that the doctor was wrong. Or perhaps that some form of alternative medicine tried in the meantime has achieved a miracle that medical science cannot explain.

If this sounds a little cynical, forgive me. Many relatives are very fair and accurate about what was said, but – even then – by the time the news has passed through a few hands, what I have described is extremely common.

A similar problem occurs when the chance of cure is much better than a small chance. Let's say a 50:50 chance. Many people find this sort of statement difficult to grasp – or at least difficult to live with. Quite often they seem to think that the doctor knows what is going to happen but doesn't want to reveal this, or doesn't want to be later proved wrong, so pretends that the outlook is more doubtful than it really is (*see* page xi).

After giving a prognosis of this kind it's especially valuable to ask the question, 'If a friend asks you what I've said, what will you tell them?'

Relative *(to GP)*: *The consultant told me that my husband has only three months to live.*

GP *(who has learned not to accept such statements at face value, but to ask for more details)*: *Can you remember what led up to him saying that? What was it you asked him? How did he reply?*

Relative: *He said it was very serious because cure was unlikely. So I asked if he might have only two or three months to live. And he said that, yes, that was unfortunately a possibility.*

GP: *Did he add anything else?*

Relative: *Well, yes, he did say something to the effect that he could live a lot longer than that, but – as you can imagine – all I could think about was this terrible news that he might have only two or three months to live.*

Note that this second version of what was said, though clearly more accurate than the first, doesn't have the same dramatic impact. It's the first version – the misleading one – that's likely to be circulating among friends and neighbours.

In general, avoid mentioning any average time, because this is so often quoted as if it is the maximum time expected, which of course it isn't. But if a patient is *unlikely* to live more than a few months, the phrase 'months rather than years', with no figure attached, can be useful and is less likely to be misunderstood or misquoted than most phrases.

And never forget that relatives will sometimes say to their friends, 'What the doctor *said* was... but I got the impression that what he really *meant* was... '. Realistic communication tries to allow for this possibility.

Is the situation bad enough for 'affairs to be put in order'?

The gentle reply should include:

- polite surprise that this was not done years ago, since we all know that we could at any time have a fatal accident or heart attack

- emphasis on the need to cater for *possibilities,* even when there is still a real chance of recovery. Unlike what happens in novels, 'putting affairs in order' does not mean that there is no hope, or that remaining life is likely to be very short, it just means sensible preparations for what *may* soon happen, or what might not happen for a long time.

Truthful hope

Often we need to explain that much will depend on how the patient responds to treatment in the immediate future. Or, in the case of the terminal patient (*see* Chapter 10) that the likely amount of time left will depend on whether or not some vital function continues to fail, or whether it stages a temporary recovery.

After the shock of the diagnosis there are other ways in which relatives may get the wrong impression as to the prognosis and whether or not anything effective can be done. For example, finding that a stroke is due to a secondary cancer may sometimes mean that more, rather than less, can be done to treat it than could be done if it were an ordinary stroke.

And when *some* kinds of cancer are found by the surgeon to be inoperable, the outlook – far from now being hopeless – may actually be better (after suitable treatment, such as radiotherapy) than when other kinds of cancer are operable. When this is so, it's not a bad idea to let patient and relative know this *before* the operation, rather than wait for the possible inoperability and then struggle to restore at least a measure of hope.

It's important to realize that this situation of 'very serious but certainly not hopeless' is a very common one in medicine, just as it is in many other aspects of life. With cancer, for example, the idea that the incurable case is completely unstoppable is not so. There are always a few people who do not just better than average, but *far* better than average.

At first it was said that AIDS, the immune deficiency disease that has swept the world in recent years, was completely hopeless and incurable, that all cases were terminal and so on. Now it's realized that, as with most diseases, though most may die, a few remain well for far longer than average.

And this doesn't mean, as many tend to think, that the diagnosis must have been wrong (though that possibility, no matter how unlikely, can sometimes be a useful way of giving a ray of hope). Cancer statistics, for example, don't show *all* patients dying within five years in *any* kind of cancer. The worst type of outlook is that after five years only about 5% are surviving. Note that this doesn't mean just one or two lucky people in every thousand. It's far better than that. Five per cent is not five, but *50* patients in every thousand. Put like this it doesn't sound quite so hopeless does it? What this figure means is that, though the outlook is very bad, the chances of doing well may be *a hundred or a thousand times better than the chance of a big win in a lottery.*

So why not put it like this to anxious relatives who crave for a little realistic hope? Or, to put it another way, who long for something a little more bearable than utter hopelessness. They can still choose optimism or pessimism. It's their choice. Maybe, as discussed in Chapter 5, abandoning all hope is the approach they prefer. But my point is that in no way can a one in 20 chance of doing well be called a *false* hope; there is nothing false about it.

Often it's valuable to add a mention of *just one patient* – preferably one recently seen – who had this outlook several years ago and who is still well. Statistically it's worthless; psychologically it can be very valuable. It helps relatives to appreciate that 'probably' means just that; it does *not* mean certainly. Every specialist sees many patients doing better than average – and nearly every doctor or nurse should be able at least to refer to patients that they have heard about or read about who have done exceptionally well. Just one case is enough to get rid of a feeling of hopelessness. What is said is one hundred per cent true. And, at the same time, properly done, it doesn't raise false hopes. As to confidentiality this is no problem to the specialist, who can easily ensure that nothing he says could possibly lead to identification of the patient concerned. A country GP would obviously have to be a little more careful.

After mentioning just this one patient the relative's response may indicate that no more need be said. He or she can now see that it is *not* an absolute death sentence that is being given. Others may want to know more about the actual statistics of it.

Doctor *(to student who – with the consent of the relative – has been present while a man's wife has been told that he has lung cancer)*: *Did you agree broadly with the way I told her? What criticisms do you have? Would you have done it differently?*

Student: *I don't think she realizes quite how hopeless it is. I feel it would have been better to be a bit more honest.*

Doctor: *Quite a lot of doctors would agree with you. But think about it. She knows that her husband may well die in the next few months, doesn't she? She understands that. Don't you think that she also has a right to know that the approximate 5% five-year survival means that more than one thousand of the men who get lung cancer in this country each year are alive and well five years later? I think she has a right to know that. If she chooses to abandon all hope that's up to her, but I think it helps most people to cope if they know that the situation is not completely hopeless.*

Do relatives, as well as patients, sometimes need protection?

Do relatives always need to be told of every complication that has developed or of every fear that the doctor has about what may be going to happen? The closely questioning attitude of some relatives means that to keep anything from them would be a mistake. But for many experienced health workers other cases can be decided on their merits without any rigid rules. For *some* distressed relatives, there seems no need to mention *all* that's known, or *all* the uncertainties, or *all* the options.

For example, if a desperately upset elderly mother is told that her son now has incurable secondary cancer deposits in his liver, she does not *have* to be told immediately (or even ever) that there are also secondary deposits in his brain. What's the point? Why make her nightmare even worse? She may well have a 'right to know', but before we become the prisoners of such slogans, would it not be better to use the sort of common sense that has been passed down the ages – and show a little restraint. Experience shows that such flexibility need not be short-sighted and need not endanger trust.

Finally, although not enough explanation is a common mistake, too much explanation can also cause confusion. Too much detail can obscure and muddle whatever vital message it is wished to convey. This isn't paternalism; it's realism.

The family doctor and the specialist

Sometimes the relative may 'phone the GP before he has any report from the hospital which can be very frustrating. This problem has been discussed in Chapter 3.

It goes without saying that as far as is compatible with truth and sincerity, the hospital doctor should aim to give both patient and relative maximum confidence in the family doctor – and the latter should do the same when speaking of a specialist.

> **One advantage of the specialist giving the bad news is that with an uncommon condition – uncommon to the doctor not specializing in it – the more cases seen, the easier it is to give some truthful hope. The GP may have seen only four previous cases, all of whom did badly. The specialist may have seen 40 cases, eight of whom did very well. Statistically their experience has been the same (the specialist's experience may well have included four consecutive patients who did badly), but it's difficult for a doctor not to be excessively pessimistic if his only experience has been of failure.**

No doubt the family doctor may need to add important points later and maybe amend what has been said.

Often the family doctor gets the impression that, in the hospital, communicating diagnosis and prognosis was done badly, or not at all. Sadly, this may be all too true. But quite frequently this is not so. One possible reason is that shock prevented the relative taking in what was said.

Another reason is that many relatives want to hear it all again – partly to see if the stories are the same. It's not easy for them to say, 'They explained everything at the hospital, but I'd like to hear it all again from you.' So they may say that little or nothing was said to them, when this is not strictly true. As with misleading first accounts of what a doctor said about diagnosis or prognosis, claims that nothing was said can sometimes be revealed to be untrue merely by asking quietly and tactfully for more details of the conversation.

When bad news is (to some extent, anyway) good news

Sometimes bad news may, in a sense, be good news. Or at least it has a good side to it, which it can be right to stress to *some* relatives, but not to others. For example, it a test shows some serious abnormality after many previous tests have been normal, it's by no means impossible that it will be privately welcomed by patient or relative, or both – and even improve their morale – for at least two reasons.

- When a relative is given a diagnosis it may be a great shock. On the other hand in a sense it may be a relief. The relief when an illness is given a name. The relief that at last investigations are to end and treatment is to begin.

- A relative who has been convinced all along, from her knowledge of the patient, that there was something seriously wrong, may now feel vindicated.

Some key points worth bearing in mind

- Inherent in some diagnostic labels are stigma, guilt, gloom and misconceptions that may be hard for the doctor or nurse to eradicate. Merely to say, 'It could have happened to me' is often helpful.

- Sometimes it's best – bearing in mind that the first thing said may be the only thing remembered and that the diagnosis may be such a shock that nothing after that is heard – to reverse the usual logical order and to give first the intention for the next week or so, then the short-term prognosis, then the long-term prognosis and only then to give the diagnosis.

- How much to say, how to say it, what words to use, how much to repeat, what to stress, what not to stress, when to stop and suggest a second interview, and many other factors, should all be heavily dependent on the relative's reaction, rather than being decided in advance. Previous experience with this particular relative (first hand or reliable second hand) will also help.

- A request to hear a little more of what was said – or not said – by another doctor will often reveal that the first version was misleading.

- When something positive is said (for example, mentioning – with complete truth – just one other patient in the same situation who did surprisingly well) it can either be said with such warmth and emphasis that it gives a great boost to morale – or so feebly and ineffectively that it does nothing and the relative feels that it is just a pathetic attempt to cheer her up.

- As with patients what is right for some relatives is wrong for others.

- For many relatives, unless a real effort is made to get across a *true impression,* such very different statements as 'possibly' only a few months and 'probably' only a few months to live are the same thing. Both are a death sentence.

- The greatest error is to think that when the outlook is bad the choice is between telling the terrible truth or being untruthful in order to shield a person from depression and hopelessness. There are always *truthful* ways to give at least a measure of hope and a boost to morale.

- In what I have called the third way of giving bad news the seriousness of the situation is not concealed, but from the very start there is a) a sensitive blending of practical and positive statements with the bad news and b) modification and emphasis of various kinds based on feedback from each individual being interviewed. Properly done, this usually means for the relative less shock, fewer tears, more real listening to what is being said and a better understanding of the situation.

Reference

1   Asher R (1955) Talk, tact and treatment. *Lancet.* **1**: 758–60.

Denial, optimism and uncertainty

Denial

For two reasons something must now be said about the concept of denial.

- Relatives in the role of *carer* may need help to understand the way in which the patient is using denial (*see* Chapter 7).

- Relatives in the role of *victim* may themselves exhibit denial, and this will affect how the doctor talks to them and helps them (*see* Chapter 8).

A person showing 'denial':

- takes a less serious view of what is happening to himself (or occasionally to his partner) than he would do if it was happening to someone else

- will not accept (or else 'forgets') what he has been told about diagnosis or prognosis

- blots out of his mind some unpleasant possibility of which he was once well aware.

Denial – whether weak or strong – is a common defence mechanism, providing protection against a situation that, at least for the moment, is a little too hard for a person to bear. Like the opposite emotion of excessive anxiety, denial can occur in people of high intelligence, who – on a purely intellectual level – would not show either. Each is seen quite commonly when the patient is a doctor, a scientist or a statistician. And as pointed out more than 30 years ago by Aldrich, denial may be just as common, perhaps even more so, in those with a strong personality and a successful career.[1]

Denial is not an all-or-none phenomenon. It may vary greatly from month to month, or even in the course of a single interview, or according to whom the person is speaking. A patient or relative may show it either when things are going well, or when they are going badly. Denial may also take

> **Relative**: *I can't understand it, doctor, my husband is an intelligent man; he was told exactly what's wrong and how serious the position is. Yet now he talks as if he had never been told anything. Does this mean that the cancer has spread to his brain?*
>
> **Doctor**: *No, it's not that. It's quite common. It's sometimes called 'denial'. It's a sort of protective mechanism. I wouldn't disturb it. Not at the moment, anyway. Some very successful people like your husband react in this way. It's not a sign of weakness. Unless you think there is some important reason to steer him back to a more realistic attitude, I'd leave it alone. It may change. Each day be guided not by what he once said, but by his current mood. We can talk about this again some time. Let me know how things develop ...*

several forms. For example, several months after accepting that they have probably not got long to live, patients may ask 'Will I always have this trouble?' The same kind of partial denial is sometimes echoed by relatives.

For many observers denial in another person is hard to understand and is therefore brushed under the carpet. This applies not just to the media, to most writers of novels and biographies, and to the general public, but also to quite a few doctors and nurses who are somewhat embarrassed by it and don't want to recognize it or talk about it.

- It is frequently distorted in the media and in the public mind by the fact that those patients or relatives who go on television (or who write or speak on the subject of their serious illness or possible forthcoming death) are obviously and inevitably those *not* using denial. The very large number of those showing it are hidden from view.

- Yet honest acceptance of the frequency of denial is vital to a true and sympathetic understanding of how some patients *and some relatives* cope with bad news.

> **Intelligent young man** *(three years after treatment for a malignant teratoma which he had clearly understood was a cancer that could recur)*: *Several life insurance companies have turned me down, but I don't believe it's because of what you treated me for. I think it's because I'm overweight.*

Some doctors and nurses, who accept the reality of denial, think that it's nearly always short sighted. They feel that it would be better for anyone showing it to be persuaded to face up to the situation and be more realistic. Others – probably the majority when the chips are down – are reluctant to interfere unless the denial seems, for some *specific* reason, to be undesirable.

If in doubt about the extent of denial, say some, why not ask the patient or relative to say exactly what is in his or her mind? The reason for not doing this is that, though it can sometimes clear the air and be welcomed, to do so risks demolishing fragile defence mechanisms that are helping a person to cope.

In the prospective study of Stephen Greer and colleagues, women with breast cancer did better if they showed either a fighting spirit or denial.[2] Patients showing *either* of these moods did better than those categorized as showing either stoic acceptance or 'feelings of hopelessness and helplessness'. Incidentally, I've always found it unattractive when patients who have done exceptionally well congratulate themselves on their fighting spirit. They would do better just to be grateful. But the media love it.

Finally, if people are at first desperately upset by bad news, but soon suppress what they have been told and show denial, does this mean that they have been poorly assessed and might have been better not told – or at least not told so much, or so bluntly, or in such an unskilled way?

Such an idea runs counter to most current thinking. At the moment the pendulum has swung more towards spelling out everything to everybody at all times. But it's at least worth considering whether those who soon show denial have not gone through a needless period of mental distress and suffering.

Doctor *(to patient after reading what another doctor had written to the GP about having 'fully informed her that effective treatment was not available')*: *Did Doctor X explain the position to you?*

Patient: *Well…not really.*

Optimism – advantages and disadvantages

Some doctors tend to avoid optimism because they fear that it may rob them of a reputation for always being totally honest and truthful, and that as a result they will be less trusted. Second, they don't want to raise what they call false hopes. Third, they may be anxious to protect themselves from criticism should things go wrong.

Relatives too may prefer pessimism. In the short term it may increase sympathy, attention and the sense of drama, and in the long term it reduces the chances of being let down or disappointed.

However, though this is a controversial subject (partly due to misunderstandings as to exactly what's being advocated), it has always seemed to me that in serious illness the advantages of sincere optimism of the right kind usually outweigh any disadvantages.

- Many relatives can be truthfully told that though a situation is very serious, it's not hopeless, the reason being that there are nearly always a few patients who do not just better than average, but *far* better than average.

- Nothing can make the position less than serious. Nothing can be promised. But the patient could turn out to be one of the lucky few. If a few patients do well, does the relative not have a right to be told this?

- The right kind of optimism suggests continued interest and continued effort. Everyone tries harder. Effort is nourished by hope. Pessimism can so easily imply that the doctor has lost interest and that anything from now on will be at best half hearted.

- Optimism usually improves quality of life, as discussed in Chapter 6.

- There should be no need to go to 'alternative' medicine in order to get support, interest, hope and optimism.

> **Patient *(energetic Managing Director, aged 56, when advised radiotherapy for rectal cancer, recurrent only four months after surgery, which was a great disappointment to those treating him)*:** *The operation was a success, so I don't see any reason why the radiotherapy shouldn't be...*

If a relative is clearly hungry for optimism, it can always be given in a truthful way. For example, doctors tend to think of 80% five-year survival as a very good prognosis and of 80% dead within five years as a very bad prognosis. But in both cases how patients and relatives feel about it will depend to a great extent on where the emphasis is placed.

- In *both* cases there is plenty of hope for those individuals who want hope, since even in the *bad* prognosis group, out of every thousand there will be 200 five-year survivors.

- In *both* cases there will also be plenty to worry about for those who can't stop worrying, since even in the *good* prognosis group there will be no fewer than 200 out of every thousand dying within five years.

The art of sincere optimism

- It's impossible to give a prognosis without colouring it to some extent with either optimism or with pessimism.

- Pessimists – whether lay or professional – may claim they are just being honest but in fact pessimism is often misleading or incomplete.

- Some relatives, like some patients, need more optimism than others. If they don't get a lot of optimism, they will be *needlessly* gloomy. With others it may be better to be very sparing with the optimism. In the middle are the majority, who in my view often don't get as much optimism as they should.

- Something said that is of no help to a patient or relative not exhibiting denial can be of great help to someone doing so. So it's often best, quietly and tactfully, to fit the amount of optimism to the amount of denial.

- Judicious use of the powerful psychological weapon of 'suggestion' can still further boost the optimism that may already have been helped by denial, thus improving quality of life still further. As suggested in Chapter 2, this is probably not done enough in mainstream medicine. But it must *not* be overdone.

- Whether at diagnosis or at relapse, relatives may need to be ready for the worst that could happen – but this doesn't mean that they have to be subjected to unrelieved pessimism. 'Hope for the best, but be prepared for the worst' is a good motto for some relatives, but not for others as they interpret it in too pessimistic a light.

- I never knew a patient or relative to be disappointed by *'I can't promise, but what we are hoping is…'*. ('Of course, you can't promise', they often say, 'we understand that – but you have given us some real hope and that makes life so much easier'.)

- Pessimistic relatives may need to be 'warned' that the patient will not necessarily do as badly as they think! The holiday that they prefer not to think about, convinced that it will never come about, may after all be possible.

- When the outlook is so bad that there's little or no room for optimism of this kind, it's usually still possible to be positive and optimistic about the goal of symptom relief.

Is optimism short sighted? Is a glimmer of hope a false hope? Excessive optimism is an obvious danger, but I feel that some hospital and family doctors are too concerned about this – and that optimism, like denial, should generally be curbed only if some specific reason can be given as to why it would be harmful.

Doctor *(to Catholic priest with lung cancer, dying, weak and wasted – after reading the referral letter, which said, 'He has been told the correct underlying diagnosis as he specifically requested to know – and subsequently seemed happier')*: *What did they tell you at the hospital?*

Priest: *They told me it was some kind of tumour, but they gave me no idea whether it was serious or not. Anyway, I'm not worrying…*

Will optimism lead to bitterness and loss of trust if things turn out badly? Many doctors fear this. But provided the optimism was given sincerely – and especially if followed by sustained friendly interest in progress – doctor and relatives now share the same disappointment: 'We know how much you yourself hoped it would *not* turn out like this', they may say.

What might be called *indirect* optimism is useful for building up morale, maximum peace of mind and quality of life. For example:

- 'However well things are going, we like to see someone like your wife at least once or twice a year for a few years.'

- 'Where do you and your husband usually like to go on holiday? France? Which part? Will you go there this summer, if he's well enough?'

For some doctors, if there is a probability that the patient has only a short time to live, such comments are insincere or somehow in bad taste. But – provided the relative has previously been told what is more likely – is what is said not truthful hope based on truthful possibilities?

At the same time it must be stressed that it would be a mistake to talk like this to those who really do prefer pessimism. Pessimism is wrong for the optimist, but optimism can be irritating to the inveterate pessimist.

Whether talking to patient and relative separately or together, before explaining the advantages of optimism, it's sometimes useful to stress that they have a *choice*. And perhaps to ask them:

- 'Have you two ever faced before the possibility that one of you might not be going to recover? If so, what was your mood? How did you cope? With optimism, with pessimism or with just a sort of neutral fatalism?

- 'In general, in *non*-medical situations, do you as a couple prefer optimism? Or pessimism? Or does one of you lean one way, one the other?'

It can put a considerable strain on a partnership if one is very optimistic, the other very pessimistic, but if that's how they have been with previous problems and crises, then when serious illness comes to one of them it may perhaps not matter so much.

Those relatives who are tempted (just as some doctors are) to offer the patient exaggerated, insincere optimism must be persuaded that this is just as big a mistake as excessive pessimism.

The same people – they may be relatives or doctors – sometimes make another mistake. They seek refuge in telling the patient that his problems are due not to his disease, but to the treatment given, though they know this is not really so. This can undermine trust in the doctor who advised or carried out the treatment concerned and is seldom, if ever, justified.

Finally, there may be some doctors who will always be more suited to pessimism than to optimism. Their personality does not fit easily into the art of sincere optimism. Often, in my experience, if they try it, they overdo it. But relatives who see such doctors may be robbed of something that can significantly reduce fear and improve quality of life – and not just in the short term.

> **Sir Peter Medawar** *(distinguished immunologist, famed for his clear thinking and forthright style, describing in his autobiography his severe stroke at the age of 54)*: *I had considered and dismissed the possibility of dying...*

Uncertainty

Uncertainty about *what to expect in the immediate future* is always to be avoided as much as possible. It can be as bad for relatives as for patients. How many more tests will there be before treatment begins? When will there be a definite plan? When is something going to be done about, for example, the patient's headache – which nobody seems interested in because they don't think it's anything to do with the main problem?

But uncertainty about *long-term* prognosis can be an ally, taking away fear because the patient can be truthfully reminded that a certain amount of uncertainty is *normal* and shared with everyone else their age, especially if no longer young. Nobody, absolutely nobody, knows whether or not they will still be alive in five years time.

With the help of optimism uncertainty becomes a source of hope rather than fear. 'Your position now', I have said to many elderly patients, 'is not really so different from what it was before you were found to have this trouble.' A variant of this would be to stress that it's not so very different to that of any one else in the community their age.

In fact, for the relative as well as the patient, anything helps that bridges the gap between, on the one hand, victims of some misfortune with an uncertain outlook and, on the other, the dangers faced by so-called normal healthy people their age. Reduce the gap. Be as optimistic as possible about the patient – and as gloomy as possible about these people who think they are normal and healthy (little knowing what waits for them just around the corner).

> **But here I must add that whereas many relatives show clearly how helpful they find this way of looking at things, there are always others who are unhappy with anything that makes the situation less dramatic. It shows clearly on their faces. The story to be passed on to friends and neighbours is robbed of some of its horror and excitement.**

To compensate for this it's only fair to give this kind of relative as much drama as possible. For example, if nothing very dramatic happened in the course of major surgery on their partner or parent or child, why not fall back on one or more serious complications that might have happened but didn't? Such consolation for stress and anxiety is always available for those whom it suits!

Extract from letter to GP (which he read out to patient's husband) from Surgeon X, always kind and caring, but often excessively pessimistic:

This appears to be a fairly solitary secondary deposit from her breast cancer …I have ordered a lumbosacral support for her…it is clear that she will continue to have some pain, which unfortunately will increase with time.

In contrast, this is what Doctor Y wrote about the same patient when he saw her a week later:

Though this recurrence is a great blow after she was doing so well, I have explained to her husband that there is a very good chance that radiotherapy (which does not usually cause any side-effects in this situation) will abolish her pain so completely that she won't need to wear the lumbosacral support given to her and will be able to resume normal activities. Many patients in this situation enjoy a good quality of life for many months, even years, so I hope the family will not start cancelling holidays or anything like that. I've strongly advised them against it.

Note that this second letter to the GP is not only far less pessimistic, but paints a picture that I would say was *more* rather than less, truthful. The first letter was meant to be honest and to face the facts, but it was actually misleading as to how much could be done.

Some brief reminders

- We may need to explain to a patient's partner or relative that *denial* is a common protective mechanism that helps many people to cope. And that it may vary from month to month – even from day to day.

- It's not always wise to try and get rid of denial. It may be better to 'allow' some patients and some relatives to practise at least a degree of it, with dignity and without loss of self-respect.

- Pessimists don't have a monopoly of truth. Far from it. It's usually not difficult for a sensitive doctor or nurse to tell how much truthful optimism each relative wants and needs.

- The right kind of optimism can improve quality of life. And the greatest advantage of all may be that it suggests continued interest and effort.

- Provided that the optimism is sincere, then – *no matter how badly things turn out* – many relatives will still be thankful for the hope they were given. Everything depends on how it's done. Optimism without promises is the key.

- Uncertainty is not a problem to fatalists but can be distressing to those increasing numbers of people who can't seem to face it. It may sometimes be possible to help them to accept what they can't change. For example, by reminding them that uncertainty is a part of life for us all, even though not to anything like the extent it used to be, following the eradication of so many forms of premature death.

No doctor has a right to be a pessimist. If you are conscious of that temperament you should fly the profession. A reasoned optimism is essential for a doctor. He must believe the best, and so he goes half way to effecting it.

Arthur Conan Doyle (medically qualified before he wrote the Sherlock Holmes Stories) speaking at St Mary's Hospital, London in 1910.

Be optimistic whenever possible...the reassuring prognosis is not incompatible with intellectual honesty.

John Ryle, Physician, Guy's Hospital 1919–35.

References

1   Aldrich G K (1963) The dying patient's grief. *Journal of the American Medical Association.* **184**: 1329–31.

2   Greer S, Morris T, Pettingale K W (1990) Psychological response to breast cancer: effect on outcome. *Lancet.* **2**: 785–7. (*See also* their letter to *Lancet* **335**: 49–50, 1990.)

Remedies, remissions and relapses

Treatments and remedies

Sometimes several *options* are first discussed – perhaps with patient and relative together – and this may be important. But often it's not sensible to complicate things too much in this way. If patient and relative know and like a doctor – or know something of the doctor's reputation – they may decide (as they might in any walk of life, medical or non-medical) to accept a professionally preferred option, rather than attempt to weigh all the evidence themselves.

Any competent doctor, having grasped what the problem is – and what the hopes and fears of the patient and relative are – knows that an ability to weigh pros and cons in the patient's best interest is part of his or her job. Good judgement – based on experience and a trained mind and making full allowance for variations in the needs and aspirations of different individuals – may be just as important as knowledge or skill.

And, of course, after hearing a specialist's advice, some will prefer to discuss it with their GP before coming to a final decision.

Next, having decided that the condition is one in which something can at least be tried, a good question to start off with is, 'Could I ask whether you have ever known anyone who has had this treatment? Have you read anything about it? Or heard anything about it?' Though often given low priority or omitted completely, such questions are just as useful when treatment is discussed as they are when the diagnosis is given. It may even save time in the long run, as it will colour what is said – and what need not be said – about the treatment. And it gives a chance to nip in the bud any obvious misconceptions. For example, it's not uncommon for relatives to say that they are strongly against a patient having a particular treatment (perhaps she is their elderly mother and in poor mental and physical condition), and their reasons turn out to be based on a false idea of what is involved.

The anxious relative will then usually need to be told more about the proposed treatments or remedies:

- what it's hoped they will achieve

- what they can't be expected to achieve

- any important risks or side-effects.

Cost will also sometimes need to be discussed.

Doctor *(after seeing a married couple together, one of them having a serious cancer but with a better than 50:50 chance of cure)*: *OK then. That sums up the position. We start treatment on Monday. Keep your fingers crossed.*

Couple: *We will. And thanks for explaining everything.*

Doctor: *Not at all. It helps if you know the plan of action. But there's one thing that puzzles me. How come you two have grandchildren? You must have been very young when you started a family.*

Both *(smiling)*: *We were.*

Doctor *(as he shakes hands with them both)*: *Are you going to watch the football this afternoon? My wife and I are hoping to see it...*

Clinical judgement – risking doing more harm than good

With some serious medical conditions, for example heart conditions, nearly everyone accepts that there can be little or no hope of cure, that sooner or later there will be further trouble, yet the ugly word 'incurable' is not usually used. With others, either the word incurable is used – or an attempt at cure is expected.

With *some* kinds of cancer, the best thing may be neither to make an attempt to cure, nor to 'give up the fight', but to handle the situation more in the way that, say, heart and blood pressure problems are treated – gently and calmly over the course of many months or years. In other words, if the chance of cure is small and any curative treatment likely to be drastic, it may be best just to help the patient towards a good quality of life, rather than risk making 'the treatment worse than the disease'.

Two ways of giving the same unwelcome news. Both are truthful, but they have very different effects on the relatives.

Doctor X, kind, but grim, unsmiling and merely anxious to be 'completely honest':

'I'm afraid it's bad news. The blood count has fallen and that means your wife can't have the full treatment. It would be too dangerous.'

That's all. Nothing positive. Nothing to indicate what happens next. Relative deeply upset.

Now Doctor Y. And note that what he says is just as sincere (though an actor could easily make the very same words sound insincere), but there is a different emphasis:

'Sit down, Mr Jayson...terrible weather, isn't it? You remember how I explained that too much of this treatment was as bad as too little – and that the blood count would tell us the best dose to give? Well, your wife's blood count is through and it shows we have given enough for the present.

'In some ways we would have liked to have given a higher dose, but at least we have not made the mistake of giving too much. And I expect you'll both be pleased that she's going home sooner than expected.

'Incidentally, I see that you live in Cartlands Road; what's happened to that pub on the corner? I used to go there when I was a medical student...'

Note that:

- Doctor Y, though disappointed with the blood count, doesn't regard it as such bad news as Doctor X does, because in general he seldom believes that exact dose and timing of drugs is quite so critical

- to another relative he might have expressed the situation differently, with more stress on the fact that this was not good news. But he knows from previous experience that this particular relative is one of those people who is liable to be plunged into excessive gloom by the slightest disappointment or setback

- the way he handles the situation is very similar to what most people expect of a good leader, or the captain of a ship, in a non-medical crisis. Keeping up morale by being as positive and unafraid as possible, within the constraints of truth.

This is neither cure nor palliation, but something in between. Much cancer care has always been of this kind, but most public and media comment ignores it. No wonder many relatives will be puzzled unless it is explained to them.

On the other hand, we may sometimes urge drastic, risky or unpleasant treatment, *because the outlook is so grim if it's not given and because we've seen it more than once to be successful*. Later, if the patient does well, both patient and relative may say how glad they are that they decided to take our advice, even though they had grave doubts about it at the time.

What everyone, patient and relative alike, wants is what gives the *best chance of benefit* with the *smallest chance of harm*. We will never get it right every time. And we will never know for sure how things would have turned out had we taken a different decision or given different advice.

Warning relatives of possible side-effects

To warn relatives as well as patients (or occasionally *instead* of patients) of possible side-effects can be very important, but – as with so many other things – a sensible balance has to be struck at some point between:

- not saying enough
- saying too much.

It certainly protects the doctor from criticism and litigation to list all possible side-effects. Then neither patient nor relative can say they were not warned.
    However:

- it's what is best for the patient and relative that counts, not what protects the doctor; and though there is no doubt that some patients and some relatives benefit from almost unlimited information of this kind, many others can be harmed and confused by it

- some side-effects will only affect a very few patients. In spite of our best efforts, certain relatives – after being told this – will go away thinking that some remote possibility is quite likely to occur. As when giving relatives the diagnosis and prognosis (*see* Chapter 4), they are told the truth, but they are left not with a *truthful* impression but with a *false* one.

- if *all* side-effects are predicted, including very remote but very serious ones, constant fear can damage the quality of life of the patient or relative who is told about them – and who perhaps almost daily expects them

- with less serious side-effects so strong is the power of 'suggestion' and the ability of the mind to affect the body that there may actually be an *increase* in side-effects, partly due to the fact that the sort of trivial symptoms that many of us get all the time (if we think about them) are now thought to be side-effects. Once again, quality of life suffers.

Nearly 40 years ago one hundred Edinburgh nurses were asked whether they would be willing to compare the side-effects of different brands of iron tablets. What they were *not* told (in those days temporary deception was thought to be acceptable when no harm could result) was that, though most were being given iron tablets of one kind or another, one of the so-called brands of iron tablet did not actually contain any iron at all. Many who thought they were taking iron, but were not, then reported exactly the same side-effects that they reported after taking iron.

Sometimes such considerations can be explained to relatives – who may well not have appreciated before how valid they are, and who may now agree that it might be kinder and wiser not to discuss with every patient all possible side-effects.

Randomizing treatment

When it is carefully explained to anxious relatives that nobody knows which of two equally suitable treatments is best – and that to randomize treatment is the best way (some would say the only reliable way) to find out – many accept this as reasonable, but some will be puzzled and disturbed because they are totally unprepared for it.

Ironically, emphasis on randomization as a *research* technique – carried out in order to advance scientific knowledge – has probably delayed its acceptance as the best way to compare the results of different policies in a purely pragmatic way. As stressed more than 40 years ago, comparing results in this way can answer *practical* questions, and thus provide future patients and their doctors with reasonably reliable information regarding the advantages and disadvantages of different policies.

Where there is no significant difference in results the more drastic or more expensive option can be given up. Many serious mistakes made by mainstream medicine this century (quite apart from earlier) could have been avoided had this been done.

When patients are being invited to become part of such a study explain this to their relatives, emphasizing that:

- randomizing gives the best chance of getting rid of bias and of having two groups that are alike apart from how they are treated, thus making false conclusions less likely

- cure rates, recurrence rates, survival time, side-effects, quality of life – or just how well patients feel (mentally and physically) – can all now be reliably compared

- such comparisons may be needed not just for new treatments, but also for standard treatments – perhaps in use for years but never before formally compared.

Fringe (complementary, alternative, natural, holistic) medicine

At the end of the twentieth century we find ourselves in a wave of enthusiasm sweeping the Western world for unconventional medicine (meaning anything not usually taught in medical schools), and relatives may enquire about this. If they don't think of it immediately, something of the kind may be suggested by a neighbour, friend or relation. If everyone is talking about something, many will want to try it. And for some the mere fact that something is not taught or approved by what critics love to call the medical establishment will give it added piquancy and appeal. In the past such waves of interest have sooner or later subsided. As in mainstream medicine, really effective remedies don't go out of fashion unless something better comes along.

There may currently be some doctors and nurses who have much the same belief in one or more of these remedies, however mystical they are, as have their patients. For the health workers who don't share this view, it will often seem best *not* to express any criticism or to say anything to reduce the faith of the patient and relative in the unconventional treatment – provided that it's not being given as an alternative to something more effective.

But sometimes relatives, as well as patients, will want a full discussion and it may be justifiable to stress:

- that mainstream medicine is not based on any particular belief or system, but on a wish to use any effective form of therapy, even when how it works is not fully understood

- that mainstream medicine fully recognizes the importance in many conditions of psychological factors and of treating the whole patient and not just the disease

- that since surprises or 'miracles' – when a patient does much better than expected (which usually just means much better than average) – are often seen in mainstream medicine, their occurrence after unconventional treatment (whether given on its own or added to conventional treatment) is without significance unless shown in reliable comparisons to occur more often than after conventional treatment by itself.

Many kinds of unconventional treatment – even if most of us don't like the aura of magic and fanciful theories that surrounds so many of them (since this suggests a backward step to ancient superstitions rather than going forwards to more progress and problem solving) – have effects that everyone must approve of, mainstream medicine itself frequently including them in its aims:

- relaxation (mental and physical, the two being closely related)

- diversion and distraction of various kinds

- hope, encouragement, positive thinking and 'suggestion'

- mood elevation, whether from psychotherapy or from appropriate medicines.

Another factor is that present generations seem less willing to accept misfortune as a normal part of life. So when the truth is that the *cause* of an illness or disability is unknown, then to offer one – as is so often done by practitioners of alternative medicine – may be very welcome to patients and perhaps to their relatives. The disadvantage of this is that by offering certain unsubstantiated theories about illness – for example that cancer is due to wrong attitudes or wrong relationships – a damaging sense of guilt may be induced, making quality of life not better, but worse.

Any kind of alternative or complementary medicine also comforts those who desperately want to feel to some extent 'in control' – and who hate the idea of just hoping for the best, following conventional treatment.

Finally, it seems rather common in fringe medicine (as in many religious cults) for the therapist to develop close and intense relationships with patients of a kind that *excludes their relatives,* thus endangering everything that the present book stands for.

> **Doctor** *(to anxious relative)*: *I can't promise anything, I'm afraid, but after two patients who responded well, we had six who didn't, so we think we are about due for another response – let's hope it will be your husband...*

Rehabilitation

For various reasons, following a serious diagnosis, many patients don't return to as normal a life as they could do. They fail, as some of them put it, 'to rejoin the human race'. Relatives can either *help* or *hinder* this aim. Rehabilitation after a stroke, for example, has been found in special studies to be less successful when the spouse is depressed, and less effective after myocardial infarction when the relatives fail to retain medical advice about resuming activity.

It's usually best that there should be an immediate plan and realistic short-term goals of some kind, even if it's only looking a week or two ahead. For example, after major surgery or any treatment where a remission is hoped for, it may make a big difference to the aim of good rehabilitation if the hospital doctor expresses some clear goal, hope or expectation to be aimed at, such as an approximate date when getting back to work or taking an overseas trip should be possible. This aim or expectation should be communicated in as positive a way as possible:

- to the patient
- to the nearest relative
- to the GP.

If life is not to be needlessly restricted there is often a need for detailed positive advice and encouragement of other kinds. For example, in the case of an elderly married couple:

- gradually get back to as full and normal a life together as possible
- why not plan your usual holiday and hope that you will both be fit enough for it?
- go round to your local pub together, if that is your custom, as often as you like. Alcohol will not do any harm provided you are sensible

- have your grandchildren to stay as usual – and, if they like climbing into your bed in the morning, that's fine, they won't catch anything. (Note that, unless this is said, even relatives who know that there is *probably* no risk, may forbid it, just to be on the safe side, which is a great shame.)

Note the use of 'both' in the second example. Be careful about possible misinterpretation, but – especially when patient and relative are both elderly – it can be good psychology and help the patient's rehabilitation if we narrow the gap between them and avoid thinking of one them as a doomed victim and the other as normal and healthy. After all, it's not so very rare in such situations for roles to be later reversed and the elderly relative to die before the patient.

Relative: *What shall I say to my husband when he asks what you told me?*

Doctor: *It's up to you, but I think I'd just say that I explained to you, as I did to him, the ways in which he is making good progress and the ways in which we are still disappointed by the lack of any progress so far.*

Relative: *Is he doing as well as you expected?*

Doctor: *Considering how ill he was a week ago, I would say he's actually doing better than I expected, but the situation is still very serious.*

Possible disadvantages of a positive, optimistic attitude at this stage include the following.

A balance has to be struck between, on the one hand, the power of optimism and 'suggestion' to speed recovery, and on the other, the risk that the patient (hopefully soon to become more of an ex-patient) loses confidence because goals are not reached.

Some doctors, especially some GPs (hospital doctors are in a much easier, more protected position) may be concerned that, should a patient be taken ill while on holiday, they may be blamed by the relative for approving it.

Finally, the morale of some patients – and sometimes even more of some relatives – seems to be helped, rather than harmed, by restrictions and rules. Perhaps this is:

- because they need to feel they are doing something to be 'in control'

- because of the way in which routines and rituals can stabilize and comfort some people and help them to cope.

In other words, whereas most patients and relatives seem to do best with as few restrictions as possible, others almost seem to need them.

Some other points:

- With an elderly patient living alone, it's important after the initial bad news – or later if relapse occurs – that the family should not assume that the patient will never again be able to live alone. It may be so. But it may not. Property should not be sold or vacated prematurely. This is a common mistake.

- As on many other occasions discussed in this book, medical social workers may be especially helpful, giving the relatives practical, psychological and financial advice.

- Some relatives, especially parents, may need to be tactfully urged not to neglect other members of the family. In the interests of good family relationships, present and future, those who are *not* ill may occasionally need extra love and attention.

- After extensive surgery – especially if affecting speech, appearance, body image, eating or bowel or bladder function – every carer, lay or professional, needs to be interested in every local problem that arises, especially in anything of an embarrassing nature. All must be happy to be close to the patient, to touch and to hold, and not be repelled either by what they see or by odours. Sometimes the doctor needs to stress the importance of this to the relative. Sometimes the doctor learns from the good example set by a nurse or a relative.

- Patient and partner, whatever their ages, may worry about whether there is any kind of sexual activity that they ought now to avoid – for example following surgery or radiotherapy for cancer in the pelvic region. If there seems no harm in it, then – without necessarily embarrassing either of them with any questions – why not reassure them by briefly saying something like this:

    'I don't want to pry into private and personal matters, but if you and your partner are normally inclined to any sexual activity or to intimate physical contact of any kind, just go ahead; it will do no harm. And if you want to talk to me – or to another doctor or to one of the

*senior nurses – about this at any time, let us know. The only reason
for my bringing it up is that some people worry about it, but are too
shy to say anything.'*

Quality of life

The aim of rehabilitation is the best possible quality of life. Relatives must
be urged not to be overprotective. Quality of life suffers when activity is not
encouraged – or, worse still, is forbidden – simply because recurrence could
take place at any time.

Sometimes, if there is a spare moment, it may be worth discussing with
the relative how quality of life for any patient – or, indeed, any of us – in
any situation depends on:

- how well we feel – which will have both physical and psychological
  aspects

- to what extent we can do the things we would like to do

- how content we are – which will depend partly on whether we compare
  ourselves with someone better off or with someone worse off.

Perhaps also discuss with the relative that when any of us are ill, injured or
disabled (no matter what the cause) we know, if we are honest, that there can
sometimes be advantages as well as disadvantages in it for us. For example:

- sympathy, drama and being the centre of attention

- being looked after and having things done for us

- possible financial advantage (compensation, disability insurance, etc.).

The difficulty is to discuss this without sounding insensitive and unfeeling
towards someone with a serious condition ('I hope you are not suggesting
he is just imagining his symptoms'), but there's no doubt that these factors
can sometimes delay rehabilitation.

Remissions

Take away fear and depression and what difference is there between a year
in remission and a year cured? None. For both partners – one the patient,

the other the relative – the quality of life during remission can be just as good as after cure, *apart from this one vital element of peace of mind.*

- For both patient and relative (though often one more than the other) a fear that can surface over and over again is that any new symptom is the beginning of the end. Much needless stress can be relieved whenever an experienced doctor can say (as he often can) that the symptom that worries the relative doesn't sound the least bit like recurrence. Sometimes this assurance can be given immediately over the 'phone.

- The media may report that someone has died 'after a ten-year battle against cancer', when he or she may really have been perfectly well for nine out of the ten years, not fighting anything, but just enjoying life as much as anyone else their age.

Doctor: *A lot depends on whether or not your husband responds to the treatment we are giving him. The position is serious, but it's certainly not hopeless. As a matter of fact I was just telling your husband that I saw a man only last week who three years ago was in the same position that your husband is in now. He's just got back from a holiday in the South of France, looking very fit and enjoying life. I remember him trying to face up to the fact that he might have only a few months to live. And now he's doing fine.*

I can't promise that your husband will do as well as that, but this other man was just as bad as your husband is now.

Self-help groups and associations where patient and/or relatives can meet others with the same condition

Special counselling for relatives may be particularly needed in certain conditions, for example AIDS or Alzheimer's disease. Self-help groups don't suit every patient or every relative but may be of great value. For many it's good to know that there are others with similar problems. Difficulties are shared. Practical advice and tips can be exchanged.

The other side of the coin is that, when in full remission after being treated, say for some type of cancer, the wisdom of 'remaining a patient' in this way must be questioned. It's right for some, but not for others. Each patient has a choice – whether to remain a patient (reading every possible book on the subject, attending meetings, trying ever more second opinions, ever more information, ever more treatments) or whether to become someone who was recently a patient, but is now just hoping for the best, knowing that there could be a recurrence of the trouble at any time, but not wanting to be reminded of it.

As far as peace of mind is concerned there will be, for relatives as well as patients, good days and bad days. Days of pessimism and days of optimism. Days of thinking that perhaps it's best *not* to have any hope but just to prepare for the worst. And days when it seems better to believe that somehow or other everything will turn out well, in spite of gloomy statistics or gloomy doctors.

Physically, too, for many patients there will be good days and bad days. Often for no obvious reason. And this needs to be explained to relatives.

Relapses

As with the original diagnosis, should doubts about possible recurrence be disclosed – to patient or to relative – when no symptoms are being caused? Or is it sometimes kinder and more sensible, given the devastating effects of something that may in the end turn out not to be a recurrence after all, to be at least flexible about the timing of disclosure?

Doctor: *But you've known for a long time how serious the outlook is for your wife, haven't you?*

Relative: *I suppose so, but I've managed to put it to the back of my mind. Sometimes I'm afraid I just couldn't accept it. And sometimes I just sort of forgot it.*

Doctor: *I understand. Don't worry about it. You are in good company. Many relatives have told me the same thing. There's no harm done.*

If relapse occurs, many relatives assume that the doctors and nurses *knew* it would happen sooner or later. If there had been, say a 50:50 chance that it would not happen – and if all concerned are upset and disappointed that it has – it may be surprisingly helpful to stress this to patients and relatives. Presumably this emphasis on how it had *not* been expected – how, on the contrary, it had been hoped that it would *not* happen – is helpful because it gets away from the scenario of the death sentence, the feeling of everything being out of control, the relentless march of unstoppable events and the suspicion that doctors have been less than frank.

It helps relatives if once again the options are explained to them, in particular whether or not it seems worth continuing with treatment aimed at fighting the disease, or whether it's better just to concentrate on comfort and symptom relief. The views of a sensible, caring relative who knows the patient well should not be lightly discarded, even when they run counter to the doctor's initial feelings. It's also wise to remember how these views may change. If they do, a good trusting doctor–relative relationship will often mean that those of the doctor will change, too. Perhaps quite independently, but perhaps partly in response to the changing attitude of the relative.

For example, so long as a man's wife is still hoping for a miracle, why not so far as possible join her and keep on her wavelength? You can't share the highs and lows with her unless you do. Be disappointed when she is, glad when she is, relieved when she is. And then, if her mood changes to a feeling that the man she loves is now very weary and has had enough – and so to a hope that it will soon be all over – why not stay with her and let her know that this is now how you feel, too?

Of course, the doctor cannot – and should not – go along in this way with the attitude of every relative on every occasion. It goes without saying that the views of the *patient* (whether known or considered likely from previous contact with him) will always come first. And that sometimes doctor and relative will have to agree to differ. But it's damaging to the relationship between a doctor on the one hand, and a sensible and loving 'next of kin' on the other, if they have different goals, hopes or fears.

The choice between optimism and pessimism is discussed in Chapters 4 and 5. And many couples facing the probable (but not certain) death of one of them within the next year or two try to steer a middle course, not thinking of the future, but just taking each day or each week as it comes.

Friction between patient and partner when relapse occurs can occasionally be quite distressing. Sometimes, for example, the patient does not wish to have treatment that the doctor feels will help, and the relative is upset and wants the doctor to put stronger pressure on the patient to accept the advice. Provided that neither patient nor relative are suffering from any manageable misconceptions, it's usually best in cases like this – even when the patient's views seem illogical and not in his best interest – to stop trying to persuade him.

Never hold it against the patient that he chooses *not* to accept your advice. Stress that his decision will *not* impair future relations – nor your wish to go on helping him in every possible way. And try to persuade the relative, too, to accept the situation and not argue or criticize the patient any more.

Too many doctors?

When relapse occurs it's quite common for more than one hospital doctor to be involved. And not just involved but willing, perhaps eager, to take full clinical responsibility. In such cases my view has always been that if possible they should agree, as mentioned in Chapter 2, that, no matter to what extent the patient is seen by more than one specialist, *only one* should be in the driver's seat, so to speak. There is a lot to be said for this at all times, but when relapse occurs it becomes especially important.

Patient, relative, GP and all hospital staff must know who it is. And if there is a change of leader, driver, co-ordinator, call it what you will, all must be told of the change. Not everyone agrees that this is necessary or even desirable. But if it's not done, low morale, confusion and breakdowns in communication can all too easily occur. Each consultant may assume that another is dealing with a new problem, and the relative is not sure who to turn to.

It was easier in the days when some hospital consultants were far less specialized than others. Then it was taken for granted that a general physician or a general surgeon would feel responsible in a way that other specialists wouldn't. Now there is a much greater need for one specialist to say to another, 'In view of the way things are going I think it would be best if you take over from me as the main consultant in the case. I shall be interested to hear how things go – be sure to let me know if you want me at any time.'

Key points to be communicated to the relatives

- After any necessary discussion of treatment options, what it is hoped to achieve, and possible side-effects, special attention may need to be given to such matters as randomized treatment studies or unconventional medicine.

- On completion of treatment, relatives can be a big help with rehabilitation. Urge them to aim at as normal a life as possible, not cosseting the patient too much.

- Reasonable and achievable goals should usually be set, and everyone should know what they are.

- In most cases the fewer rules and restrictions the better, but some patients and relatives seem to need them in order to feel secure.

- Special associations and self-help groups, though they don't suit everyone, can be a big help to relatives as much as to patients, and it's important that both should be made aware of them.

- Many patients and relatives are able to enjoy remissions to the full, provided that they have reasonable peace of mind. A lot will depend on the attitude to *uncertainty* (*see* Chapter 5). Fatalism helps – what will be, will be – but is currently somewhat out of fashion.

- 'Suffering from an incurable disease' or 'fighting a long battle against cancer', or similar phrases popular with the media, are often a long way from the true picture of good – or fairly good – quality of life while in remission.

- If relapse occurs, relatives may again ask about treatment options. Their views may make a contribution to whether or not to continue treatments aimed at arresting or slowing down the disease. Or whether just to concentrate on symptoms.

The relative as adviser and carer

Assessment

As mentioned in Chapter 1, in any serious situation the wise doctor, nurse, or social worker will want to assess as far as possible each relative, especially the main carer or companion.

Here are some key points to consider, assuming for the moment that the relative is a woman (daughter, mother, sister, wife or partner). The same thing, of course, applies to a key friend.

- What seems to be her psychological state? Her physical health and strength? Has she had experience of similar situations?

- Has she any particular theory or belief about the cause and nature of the condition that the patient is suffering from? Or an opinion on the best treatment? If the doctor privately doubts her theories, or even strongly disagrees with them, it may be best to bear in mind her perceptions and expectations and not reject them, at least not too bluntly.

- How good is the relationship between carer and patient? Be alert to any possibility that the carer may not always speak or act in the best interests of the patient, who may, for example, be a mother-in-law with whom relations have always been strained.

- A special problem arises when the nearest relative is an experienced doctor or nurse. Young doctors or nurses looking after the patient may find it difficult to handle this confusion of roles. They may reject helpful advice. Tact and forbearance are needed on both sides.

- Near the end of a long relationship, it may help, especially when seeing patient and relative together, to recall previous times of fear and stress, or previous crises. I'm not sure why, but it seems to help. Perhaps it serves as a reminder that if an unexpected recovery – or a narrow escape – occurred once, it could happen again.

- Ask them: 'Do you find that you cope with crises in different ways?', 'Who seems to cope best?', 'What previous experience do you have of role reversal, when one has to do the jobs normally done by the other?'

> As with most subjects, the more you think about relating to the relatives the more there is to it. Different situations. Different ages and generations. The patient may be a child, a young adult, middle aged, or elderly. The relative, too, may be any of these.
>
> The prognosis will also vary. This book is concerned only with serious or potentially serious situations, but this still allows a vast range of possibilities, both in the short term and in the long term.
>
> And note that the amount of contact that a doctor has with the patient's relatives in the course of a serious illness will vary from being quite brief to a close and warm relationship spread over many months.

Assessing the domestic situation

Bear in mind that the biggest current problem in a family, or between partners, is not necessarily the illness that concerns the doctor.

- There may be someone else in the home, perhaps disabled or very elderly, being cared for.

- There may be someone with a drink or drug problem.

- There may be serious debt or other financial problems.

- There may be constant friction of some kind.

There must be no prying for its own sake – and no undue time spent on the matter – but such information may be important should difficulties or unexpected behaviour arise and need to be understood.

Additional background information about the patient

A relative can often help the doctor or nurse to understand the patient better, adding to what the patient has said.

    For example, if the patient seems tense and anxious; and nobody knows quite why:

- the relative may sometimes be able to help the doctor to tease out the problem – perhaps a needless fear of some kind – or perhaps the relative is able to tell the doctor of a special fear that the patient has had for many years, but which he is too embarrassed to mention himself

- the relative may be able to say how the patient has reacted before to serious illness, or perhaps explain that her partner has *'always* been a worrier' or 'has *never* been able to express his feelings'. This is very useful information

- the relative may be able to tell the doctor how the patient reacted to what the doctor said to him – how well he understood it, or how much it seemed to help him.

It may be quite illuminating to compare what the relative says with what the patient says, not necessarily preferring one account to the other, but balancing the two.

Here we may need to be a little subtle. We must not seem too curious, but we may pick up clues from one relative that we would not pick up from another. If you want to know a man's secret vices, commented an astute doctor many years ago, ask his sister-in-law (mother, wife, daughters and sisters are all too loyal to say anything and other men will not want to give him away).

Note that initial assessments may sometimes later prove to be quite wide of the mark. Be prepared to make adjustments. Whether as advisers or carers, relatives sometimes surprise us by turning out to be much better (or, sadly, much worse) than we had expected.

Perhaps relations between patient and relative may turn out to be much less happy than we had first assumed. Sutherland, who has not been given sufficient credit for his pioneering psychological studies more than 40 years ago, found that the marriages of many of the cancer patients he saw were either what he called *façade* marriages or *hostile* marriages (he was not suggesting that there was anything special about cancer patients, he was just looking at the situation in the way this book does).[1]

In a *hostile* marriage a husband may appear at first as very concerned. Then his constant enquiries (as to exactly how much longer the patient may live) become a little too persistent – and it sometimes turns out that this is due not to more than average love and concern, but to the reverse. Perhaps there is a potential new partner waiting in the wings and he is getting impatient. This situation may affect what is said and what is done in the coming months, just as a *façade* marriage may affect whether or not a terminal patient is nursed at home, as discussed in Chapter 10.

Finally, in the light of the assessment, remember the following.

- Discuss once again with the relative the patient's diagnosis and prognosis to make sure that there has been no serious misunderstanding, often stressing that the prognosis may change. As mentioned in Chapter 4, even if it doesn't, discussion of a serious prognosis is seldom a matter to be dealt with once and then forgotten.

- Prepare key relatives as far as possible for what is *probably* going to happen, and perhaps for what is *possibly* going to happen. Some anxious relatives have difficulty separating the two and, for them, it may be wiser to concentrate on the probabilities and omit the possibilities.

- Even now (as when giving a prognosis at the time of diagnosis) words like 'may' and 'might' are often either forgotten or never registered ('The doctor said it would go to her lungs and that really worried me, but he was wrong, it never did').

- Predicting forthcoming symptoms and how the disease is likely to progress is far more difficult than many of the public realize. Individual variation is underestimated. Some relatives suspect, when this uncertainty is explained to them, that this is just an excuse for not revealing what the doctor knows will happen. But it's not.

- Explain to inexperienced relatives that in almost any condition, good days and bad days (or good weeks or bad weeks, or good months and bad months) are the norm. This is one of the reasons why assessing the

---

Doctor: *If you prefer just to prepare for the worst, that's entirely up to you, but I think it will help your husband – and probably give you a better life together – if you are a bit more optimistic and work away at getting back to as normal a life as possible. You are both over 70, aren't you? Well, as I say, it's entirely up to you, but now that you know that he will not necessarily get any recurrence, why not try as far as possible to live like others your age? Most people don't keep wondering what the average survival time is for people their age, do they? Or what might be the next thing they'll get wrong with them? They just get on with their life as best they can ... Let's talk about this again next week.*

value of remedies (whether mainstream or unconventional) can be so difficult.

- Some relatives are helped by a reminder that we all die, but that many of us – including those who have been diagnosed as having something that is probably not curable – will die *without* having any terminal illness. We may well be ill before we die, but only in a way that suggests that it's just a temporary setback, perhaps an episode of infection. Nobody regards it at the time as a terminal illness. Or perhaps we die suddenly without any warning, as discussed in Chapter 10.

Discussing diagnosis and prognosis

How is the relative to discuss diagnosis and prognosis with the patient? Relatives often ask for advice about this. Rather than just say, 'I don't think I can advise you on that, it's up to you', some of the various points made in other chapters of this book may need to be discussed.

There are those who think that if loving relatives beg the doctor not to tell the patient certain things about diagnosis or prognosis, it's nearly always the duty of the doctor to persuade them that this attitude is wrong. I'm not so sure. Though it's true that the doctor's first duty is to the patient, it can be a great mistake, in my view, for the doctor either to follow rigid ethical or legal rules – or to think that he or she always knows better than do loving partners or relatives. It may not be wise to try too hard to persuade them, let alone go against their wishes.

The 'denial' shown by patients may need to be discussed with relatives. Denial (*see* Chapter 5) is quite common, not only with regard to prognosis, but also in association with certain depressing or frightening symptoms, for example dementia, incontinence, blindness or paraplegia. This may puzzle and surprise some relatives and we may need to discuss it with them.

- Relatives often say – with some surprise – either that their partner has never discussed with them how serious their illness might be, or alternatively that they did once, but now talk only of possible recovery.

- Some patients show a lot of denial, but others only a little and only at certain stages of their illness.

- A patient may accept a serious outlook, then a few months later 'deny' it. Then revert to acceptance. There are no rules, no fixed pattern.

- Relatives (and staff) should be advised to base what they say to the patient on his current mood rather than on what he once seemed to accept – and still less on what it is recorded that he was once told.

- Sometimes the ambivalence that is so common in human thinking seems to allow simultaneous acceptance and denial ('I have accepted that I have a terminal illness', a patient once said to me, 'but have decided that I'm not going to die').

- Sometimes there is no real denial, but neither relative nor patient want to spell out anything embarrassing or painful, preferring to keep it to themselves. And neither of them want anyone else spelling it out either.

As with so much else, stressing that denial is common can be itself be a surprisingly big help to the relative, emphasizing that it does not mean cowardice or character weakness. The paradox here is that we admire calm and realistic acceptance of a situation, yet we may also admire those who refuse to do this. In fact we may regard this second stance not as a rather cowardly failure to face up to the facts, but as a brave refusal to admit defeat.

Patients are often pictured as 'knowing' or 'not knowing'. But a frequent situation is that though they *have not* accepted that their life is *definitely* coming to a close, they *have* accepted that it *may* be doing so. So they prepare for this possibility. Relatives may help us to understand better what is going on in the patient's mind. But what a patient is thinking about his prognosis may quite often be as much a mystery to a close and loving partner as it is to the doctor.

In some marriages or similar relationships, when one of the couple may not have long to live, the two of them discuss everything openly and frankly together. But many other couples, however close and warm their relationship, don't do this. And I'm not sure that one way is necessarily better than the other. Sometimes an important part of love and trust – whether between relative and patient, doctor and patient, or doctor and relative – is to leave things unspoken. This sensitive area is also discussed in Chapter 10.

Practical help and advice

The contribution that the caring relative can make to quality of life has been discussed in Chapter 6. Don't forget to give information about special organizations or charities. Jones and colleagues interviewed the relatives who had coped with the caring of 207 patients who had died at home of cancer.[2] Many realized later how much practical help and advice they could have had, but they didn't know it was available.

Other points to consider are:

- the supply of practical equipment for nursing in the home – and this does not refer just to specialized aids. 'A washing machine for the exhausted carer may be of more value than extra counselling', is how Barbara Monroe puts it[3]

- full demonstrations of how to use it, including *supervised practice* and *rehearsals*

- when both patient and relative are elderly and perhaps not seeing too well, clear instructions on a large card referring to the LARGE RED TABLETS or the SMALL BLUE TABLETS, written in capital letters with a black felt pen

- basic nursing techniques from a community nurse

- financial advice from a medical social worker.

Sometimes advise the carer not to give *too* much sympathy, nor to show *too* much flexibility.

'Don't sympathize with me, will you?' said a patient with advanced cancer to me once, 'It just makes me feel worse'. Explain this to relatives. Too much kindness may also make a patient feel that he has no chance whatever of recovery. 'It must be hopeless', he thinks, 'or they wouldn't be so kind to me' – when the truth is that there is still a real possibility of recovery.

A little teasing or gentle bullying, with mock strictness and threats of punishment, can be good for morale. But, as with other kinds of humour, both doctors and relatives have to be very careful or the effect will be the opposite of what they would like. The secret is to choose the right patient and the right relative, and to be guided by feedback.

As with rehabilitation after treatment (Chapter 6), whatever the outlook doctors must try to persuade carers not to make patients more inactive or helpless than they need be. Often this mistake is made out of love, but sometimes for less attractive reasons. Health workers learn to recognize a certain kind of agitated concern and anxiety (about the patient doing too much and not resting enough) that seems to spring not from love, but from the opposite.

Another kind of cosseting that, like kindness, can be overdone by relatives is to press more food on patients than they want. 'You will never feel better if you don't eat properly' may be an expression of love, but it can be very inappropriate. Rejected food is interpreted by some relatives as rejected love. All the skill and tact of a doctor or nurse may be needed to correct this common mistake, for example by stressing that the body in its present state can only handle so much food and that more than that may do harm. Other ways of expressing care and love must be found.

Relaxation and diversion

Advise the carer – if she is not well aware of it already – how relaxation (both mental and physical, the two being closely related), distraction (diversion) and any kind of mood elevation can all help pain, fear and many other symptoms, both physical and psychological.

Relaxation will include for some people meditation of various kinds. For others such things as favourite pieces of music or pictures of familiar places visited long ago, preferably with happy memories. Others may desire something more active, perhaps such creative diversions as needlework (not just for women – many men enjoy it, especially embroidery of crests and insignia), model making, jigsaw puzzles, arts and crafts. You might think that a good book could be a great consolation, but most patients find it hard to concentrate on one, unless feeling really well.

Urge relatives whenever possible:

• to give the patient a feeling that he can still be of use to others

• to give him simple – or not so simple – mental or physical jobs to do

• to ask his advice and let him feel that he is still making decisions.

Creating as normal an atmosphere as possible

Encourage relatives who are not already doing it to be as *normal* as possible. Some relatives need positive encouragement or they may think that normality is not appropriate in a serious or tragic situation.

With humour, for example, as discussed in Chapter 2, this should generally be *exactly the same* as it was when life was normal, before the blow of a serious diagnosis or before the start of pain or incapacity. Any joke worth telling before the illness is worth telling now. And in exactly the same way – not in a hushed tone, as if in church, or in a hesitant way, not quite sure if it's the right thing. Any bit of local gossip is also just as worth passing on now as

Example of quick concise note made in the medical records of a very ill man, after helpful information from a relative:

'Wife says he was born in Australia. Has been in the police since he was 20. She's in the police, too – that's how they met. Liable to nightmares for as long as she has known him. May drink fairly heavily when under stress.'

it was when the patient felt well. And in exactly the same way. No hesitancy. No apology. Just normality.

To many carers, whether or not they have experience of looking after ill people or coping with a patient's fears, all this will come naturally. Quite unselfconsciously and effortlessly – and without any advice from anyone – it will be obvious to them that this is the best way. Totally inexperienced teenage girls may make a better job of this than many mature adults. For a suffering patient, perhaps especially an elderly one, their cheerful presence, their smile and their chat may be a real tonic – pure gold in fact.

Some doctors and some relatives feel that such normality, if the patient may not have much longer to live, is not only inappropriate, but also not quite honest, a pretence that the situation is not as serious as it really is. Perhaps there is sometimes a small grain of truth in this. But in general I can't agree with it and feel sure it's a wrong view, one that is quite a common cause of patients being unhappier than they need be.

However, all this is appropriate only if the relative, like the doctor or nurse, is prepared to discuss serious matters with the patient whenever the patient wishes. Nothing is worse than for jokes or gossip to block the wish to have a serious discussion. A good carer, whether amateur or professional, should be equally comfortable with either kind of conversation.

Friction between relative and patient

If faced with anger or bitterness from the patient, the carer will need to be very forgiving. In the real world we can't expect either seriously ill patients, or those who struggle to care for them, to be saints. At least not all the time. Either can be lovable or impossible, calm or irritable, unselfish or selfish, courageous or cowardly. And sometimes all of these in a single day.

Jealousy of the good fortune and good health of the carer also needs to be regarded as understandable and to be forgiven. I recall two sisters, aged about 70, one dying. Suddenly when I was alone with the one doing the caring, she whispered to me bitterly, almost viciously, 'She always thought I would be the one to go first, now it's her and she can't forgive me for being well, when she's so ill.' Sad, but true.

The mechanism of symptoms

This might seem of little importance or interest to a distressed relative, but it can take away much of the fear of what is going on. A new symptom is not necessarily due to the main condition.

- Some symptoms may be the sort that anyone could get after a spell of being confined to bed.

- Some may be due to a complication, perhaps a treatable one.

- Some may be due to an unrelated condition.

- Some may be a side-effect of treatment, which a change in treatment may put right.

Especially in cases of cancer, any of these four possible reasons may be very welcome news for the relative, as much as for the patient. And a relative will have more confidence in a doctor who is clearly bearing in mind such possibilities.

There are other features of the patient's illness that may need to be discussed with a carer.

Some relatives will be surprised to hear that bodily (somatic) symptoms may be partly or wholly 'psychological' and associated with guilt or anxiety or depression. Everyone accepts that a headache may be emotional, but with other parts of the body many people can hardly credit it. Explain to them that chest pain for example may be psychological, as may be a feeling of shortness of breath. Hyperventilation may need to be explained to a relative, who may be able to help with its diagnosis and treatment. Nausea may be a symptom of fear or other emotional distress. So may bowel symptoms. So may loss of appetite.

Some will also benefit from an explanation of the difference between, on the one hand, feeling depressed and, on the other, suffering from a true clinical depression – the latter being a grey colourless world of deep despair,

with low self-esteem, guilty feelings over fairly trivial matters and loss of normal emotional feelings, all of these symptoms being typically worse on
waking. Explain this sort of thing to those relatives who are receptive and
interested, but – as with denial – it would be foolish and time wasting to
attempt to do so with *all* relatives.

For patients or relatives who *must* have a *physical* label and an explanation (because they feel worried or insulted by anything less) it may
occasionally be better just to offer something that they can accept, or even
just to go along with their own theories and beliefs and leave it at that.

Caring for the carer

Finally, after discussion with the carer about how the *patient* is getting on, the
doctor should ask the relative 'And now how about you, how are things going
with you? Are you looking after yourself? Are you getting enough sleep?' Don't
forget that Wilkes found that one quarter of relatives coping with the caring of
elderly patients were themselves over 70 years old.[4] But with the right kind of
encouragement, practical advice and moral support, even elderly carers may
achieve more than they would ever have thought possible. For example:

- some people need to be reassured that having less sleep than usual is
  unlikely to do them any harm

- ask them what they find the *worst* thing – the greatest stress?; this is
  always an interesting and instructive question to ask a carer

- some burdens and problems seem easier to bear when subjected to a
  little friendly sympathetic humour.

It may help a patient in a special kind of way, if a relative (perhaps a
wife or daughter) tells him, 'The doctor was saying again how relieved
she is that the X-ray is normal', or 'She admires your patience', or 'She
says that looking after you has taught her several things that will help her
with other patients'. Note that the doctor has made such comments as
much for the benefit of the patient as of the relative, being fairly confident that they will be passed on.

Carers can very easily feel not just mentally and physically exhausted, but
trapped. No life of their own, their whole existence revolving around that of

someone else. Show that you realize this, that you have at least some idea of what it must be like. For some relatives indirect ways of showing this may be more effective than saying it directly. For the relative who badly needs a break but is reluctant to take one, it may help if the doctor not only 'gives permission' for a holiday, but also 'insists' and 'orders' one – telling the *patient* that the *carer* needs this, giving reasons, seeking the patient's full co-operation and suggesting how it could be done.

When a relative is coping well, be sure to give whatever *praise* is due. These are the sorts of point that can be made. They must be sincere – and not made too often – but should be borne in mind because they can provide powerful moral support.

- 'You dealt with that last crisis very well.'

- 'You were right to call me' (relatives may contact the doctor either too much or not enough).

- 'You are doing very well for someone who has never before had to cope with this sort of situation.'

- 'He is lucky to have you looking after him. Believe me, I have seen men in the same sort of position as your husband is in now, whose wives were not nearly as determined as you are to keep going – and to do it well.'

Guilt – at least certain kinds of guilt – may be understandable and almost inevitable, for example:

- when relatives wish some old person would hurry up and die because they feel that they cannot take much more of the burden of caring for them. 'Giving permission' to feel like this can help ('I'd probably feel the same, anyone would')

- when they feel irritable with the patient – for example, after having to listen to endless self-pity – carers may need reassurance that they are only being human. Perhaps even be praised for their restraint.

Doyle[5] stresses how an exhausted relative may welcome not only 'permission' but even encouragement to express feelings of anger, guilt, jealousy, anxiety, self-pity and so on. Hopefully, their mere expression will be beneficial. But a mixture of *extreme* guilt and anger probably has some deeper underlying cause, some jealousy or dispute or deception going back many years. Psychiatric or spiritual help may be needed.

An 80-year-old woman was ready to leave hospital, but it was unlikely that she would ever again be able to live alone. She had two married sons, both living in comfortable homes and with the space to have their mother live with them, but both refusing to have her, giving no good reason, but saying it was out of the question. One had young children in the house. The other an aged father-in-law and mother-in-law living in the district. Both seemed fond of their mother. Both felt guilty about it. But neither would budge. They would not have her, even if they took it in turns, each for a few months at a time. And they did not want the matter to be discussed with their wives.

What should be the attitude to this sort of situation? Keep up maximum pressure on them, trying to find out if there is something behind it that they are not revealing? And making them feel even more guilty than they do already? Or just accept the situation and try to make other arrangements?

Reminders and useful options

- After assessing experience, perceptions, expectations and so on, it may help to discuss with relative and patient together how they have coped with previous crises or problems in their life.

- Relatives and health workers can help each other to understand the patient better. The relative may be very useful as an adviser, and if so should always be warmly thanked ('You've been a great help') at the end of an interview.

- An increasing number of patients like fairly blunt talk about the situation. These are the ones who appear on television. But there is an important group who seem to get on better either 'denying' it – or just not discussing it – and this may need to be explained and discussed with relatives.

- Relatives with no nursing experience may need plenty of help and practical instruction, including the careful rehearsal of every procedure under supervision.

- Some relatives may need advice about various ways of helping a tense, anxious or depressed patient. Relaxation (both mental and physical, the two being intimately related) may help. So may any form of diversion or distraction. So may mood elevation, psychological or pharmacological.

- The atmosphere surrounding the patient should be as normal as possible. And the patient should if possible still do something useful, however small. This will help his self-respect as well as giving him something else to think about.

- Apart from ways in which relatives can help with the task of easing symptoms of any kind, *explaining* each one to them will often help to take some of the fear out of the situation.

- Relatives may need to be watched for excessive mental or physical stress, possibly threatening breakdown, as discussed in Chapter 10. Praising their efforts will help them to keep going.

References

1   Sutherland A M (1956) Psychological impact of cancer and its therapy. *Medical Clinics of North America.* **40**: 705–20.

2   Jones R V, Hansford J, Fiske J (1993) Death from cancer at home. *BMJ.* **306**: 249–51.

3   Monroe B (1993) The Psycho-social Dimension of Palliation. In *Management of Terminal Malignant Disease,* 3rd edn (eds C Saunders and N Sykes). Edward Arnold, London.

4   Wilkes E (1989) Ethics in Terminal Care. In *Doctors' Decisions* (ed. G R Dunstan and E A Shinebourne). Oxford University Press, Oxford.

5   Doyle D (1989) Talking to the Dying Patient. In *Talking with Patients – a Basic Clinical Skill* (ed. P R Myerscough). Oxford University Press, Oxford.

The relative as victim

In every serious illness the nearest relative may be thought of not only as some-one who needs information from us, who can advise us and who may play a leading part in caring for the patient, but also as a victim needing our help. Some relatives need us hardly at all. But occasionally, especially near the end of a patient's life, a relative may justify as much of our time as does the patient.

Cicely Saunders wrote in the early days of St Christopher's Hospice, 30 years ago, 'the staff aim to open themselves to the problems of the relatives and accept their care as part of their responsibility'.[1] But how much time can be found for this in the average hospital, or even in primary care?

Relatives may ask for help, but suppose they don't? Should we invite them to express their concerns freely and thus do what a nurse that I used to work with called 'take the lid off'? May we not be opening a Pandora's box of more troubles than we can possibly find time to cope with?

Fortunately, in spite of all that is being said today about the importance of bringing everything out into the open and thoroughly discussing it, distressed relatives can often be helped in much briefer ways. Ways that don't take so much time away from patients – or from other relatives in greater need.

As with patients, so with relatives in the role of victim, we will ideally want to know something about their background, but we will need to ask for it in a rather different way:

- previous major stresses or crises?

- serious past illness, mental (be tactful) or physical?

- special friend or relative to turn to for support?

But remember that unless the relative becomes so distressed that she needs to be regarded as a patient, such enquiries should be made in an informal and sensitive way. I once heard it said of a relative at a staff meeting that 'at first he didn't want to tell us anything about his problems, but he has now become more co-operative'. It sounded a bit like a police investigation.

Needless or exaggerated fears

These are discussed in Chapters 4 and 10. Direct questioning as to exactly what it is that a relative is afraid of may clear the air, but some may rather resent being questioned in this way, as if by a parent or teacher. Sometimes it's wiser to rely on less direct methods.

If a relative makes some striking or illuminating remark about what they are afraid of, always record it in the case sheet. Just a few words in quotation marks, without any comment, is usually enough. This will serve both as a reminder to the doctor or nurse who heard it and as information for other staff. Much can be learned in this way of the hopes and fears of patients and relatives, and about the relationship between them.

What is said with the aim of *indirectly* easing the fears of a relative will depend partly on the attitude and personality of the relative, and partly on the attitude and personality of the doctor or the nurse. But just a minute or two of relaxed *'normal'*, friendly conversation is surprisingly valuable, taking away some of the nightmare quality of the situation.

Distressed relatives, as much as patients, may feel that they are locked into a world that is no longer quite real. Anything that makes them feel themselves again – perhaps a quick word about the street where they live, or their job, or their family, or what the media are currently talking about – will help. Not every time. Not with everybody. But get the timing right and it helps. Though their world may seem shattered – and their mind in turmoil – they are still the same people. They are not suddenly mere cardboard characters in a medical tragedy.

With elderly relatives, especially the very elderly, don't forget that they were young once. They have their past and their memories. Where they were born? What have they done in life? Grandchildren? What ages are they? Ask an elderly woman the price of bread or milk when she was young. How does she feel about the state of the world today? Ask a man if he played football. If so, what position on the field? How good was he? How many goals scored? In just a minute or two it shows respect and helps to take away fear.

But don't forget feedback. If there are signs of this approach not being appreciated, don't go blundering on. Rapidly switch to something more immediate and relevant.

A sense of proportion

One partner may always have tended to be the leader, the stronger in a crisis, the decision maker in financial affairs or the one responsible for keeping in touch with a scattered family. If this is the one who is now ill, the strain for the other – quite apart from fear about the diagnosis and prognosis – may be considerable. And even if such things have been more or less equally shared, the relative may feel out of his or her depth trying to cope with things normally done by the patient. It helps for the doctor to show that such difficulties, as well as the more obvious one of anxiety over the course of the illness, are appreciated.

What do you say when a distressed relative asks 'Why me?' Some have already had so much misfortune that the only possible reply is 'God knows, it just seems so unfair. I've seen very few people in my life who have had as much bad luck as you've had'. But sometimes there is a lot less justification for complaint and a doctor or nurse who has seen a lot of suffering may be thinking: 'Why *not* you? Why only others? Life never goes on for ever being a bed of roses. The human body is such a complicated piece of machinery, the real surprise is that it doesn't break down more often. Don't you think you should maybe stop feeling quite so sorry for yourself?' And just occasionally it pays to *say* this, rather than just *think* it; and the relative may later thank you.

If any blessings are to be counted, however, it's preferable for relatives to do it themselves, perhaps after a little astute steering in this direction. One

---

For the moment the time has past when it was acceptable for a family doctor just to say gruffly (as one of them was reputed to have said regularly 50 years ago), 'Remember how at your wedding you promised to keep him in sickness or in health? Well, you've had the health, this is the sickness.' At the same time it's possible, as everyone knows when a friend or relative is finding it difficult to cope, to be a little *too* sympathetic. Soft sympathy is not always the best thing for morale.

of the advantages of a patient being in a hospital ward with others is that her visitor may see other relatives visiting patients who are worse off. Relatives may be profoundly affected by this and thus feel less sorry for themselves.

Here are some other points that can sometimes be *gently* put to selected unhappy relatives (carefully watching their reaction).

- 'I can assure you there are ways in which the present position could be worse – having seen many similar cases several aspects of your wife's case are a great relief to me.'

- 'Has it ever crossed your mind that what has happened now could have happened ten years ago? Then all those good times in the last ten years that you have told me about would never have been?

- 'Don't forget that a hundred years ago there was far more death and disease in childhood and in early adult life – and therefore far more grief and tragedy – than there is today.' At least we get less of it. People living in those days would envy us.

- 'Perhaps I shouldn't say this in case it sounds unsympathetic, but do you ever stop and consider all the people who have had less happiness in their lives than you have had?'

- 'At the present time it's hard for you to bear, but – as you probably know – after going through a crisis many people say they have a deeper understanding and appreciate life more than they did before.'

But be careful. Don't overdo it. One of these points may be quite enough. With many people, it will be safer not to mention any of them. One of the reasons for saying this is that, though the person you speak to may be helped, if what is said is reported to others it can easily be made to sound insensitive and unsympathetic.

Optimism and pessimism

It sometimes helps to stress, as mentioned in Chapters 4 and 5, that relatives, like patients, have a *choice* of being either optimistic or pessimistic. And to remind them that this is true of everything in life and not just of medical matters. Some people spend all their lives preferring hope and optimism. Others prefer pessimism – they reckon they run less risk of being disappointed.

Optimism and pessimism are, in fact, two equally valid 'coping strategies', but in serious illness optimism gives *most* patients and *most* relatives a better quality of life.

- With optimism, life is more normal, more like that of everyone else.

- With pessimism, life is less likely to be normal; and the patient, instead of giving up the patient role, tends to continue in it. This can lose friends, who will probably be more willing to visit if there is a little more normality and optimism.

As with so many other things in life, there will be good days and bad days.

- When feeling optimistic ('maybe the doctors got the diagnosis wrong', 'maybe a cure will soon be found') a loving couple may plan for the future almost as if they had as much to look forward to as any other couple their age.

- When feeling pessimistic they may be overwhelmed with a feeling of sadness and heartbreak and find it difficult to fend off paralysing self-pity.

Fears for the future can be eased in various truthful ways. For example, placing emphasis on sharing an uncertain future with millions of others. As discussed in Chapter 5, to narrow the gap between 'victims' (a word that the media love, but which the 'victims' and their relatives hate) and the rest of the population, it sometimes pays to be as pessimistic as possible about so-called normal healthy people, who could at any moment be killed in a car crash or have a fatal heart attack or stroke. Why not slip in a mention of what a lot of trouble these so-called normal, healthy people cause when they die having never made a will?

Try it and watch the effect. Like every other suggestion in this book, with some relatives it will not help in the least. But with others it will. Some anxious patients and relatives – desperately worried about their uncertain future – visibly brighten up when this point is made.

There are some relatives who will be excessively pessimistic unless given more optimism than would be appropriate in someone with a more open and balanced attitude. This is another example of the fact that, in spite of all the rhetoric about total honesty and so on, the doctor or nurse working 'at the coal face' has to consider the likely

**effect of their words and not what the effect ought to be if every-
thing said was calmly weighed and considered.**

> Never forget that, just as the dry-eyed relative may really be desperately
> upset, so the apparently cheerful optimist – even the joking optimist –
> may be inwardly suffering agonies of anxiety.

Chapters 5 and 7 have discussed how we quite often need to explain the
patient's 'denial' to the relative and how, in my view, denial immediately
after bad news suggests that too much was said – or said too bluntly. The
person could not tolerate it, so nothing was achieved except a period of
intense shock and mental suffering before denial took over and suppressed
it.

Is this ever true of relatives in the role of victims? I suggest that it is. As
with the patient, those doctors who are merely relieved to be finished (as
they see it) with the painful job of giving a relative bad news may never be
aware that any denial has taken place, let alone the extent of it. But it's not
uncommon.

The alternative view to this is that the doctor must do his duty – the relative must be told everything – and it is then hardly of any concern to the
doctor if relatives 'choose' to deny what they have been told.

When the carer gets little thanks from the patient

One of the ways in which a caring relative can be a victim is as a victim of
ingratitude. Due to a change in personality, or sadly even without this, the
dying patient – instead of showing the sort of uncomplaining courage that is
so impressive – may be irritable and ungrateful.

Whereas a lifelong hypochondriac may (interestingly enough) complain
very little when seriously ill, a man with a reputation for being kind to others may say hurtful things to the wife caring for him in his terminal illness.
In contrast to this – and as an example of the sort of light relief that health
staff badly need sometimes – Derek Doyle gives an example of the opposite
change. A dying man became so considerate and generous to his wife that
she exclaimed, 'how can he be so charming now, after the way he has
treated me for the last 30 years?'[2]

Another problem is that some relatives get very little sympathy or support from other relatives. Sometimes they get irritable with each other. Perhaps each can be tactfully urged to give the other more understanding.

Role reversal

When the relative appears mainly in the role of victim – perhaps for a time suffering more than the patient – there may be a reversal of roles, with the *patient* helping doctors and nurses to understand the *relative* better. Here is where the sensible, loving patient may be able to help the doctor to care for the relative! Quite apart from the value of the advice it can be an excellent thing for the patient's morale to be consulted in this way.

For example, if a relative is very distraught, it may be helpful for doctors and nurses to hear from the patient whether he or she is often like this, easily upset and depressed. Or whether, on the other hand, it's out of character. If there's nothing very new about it, the needs of other relatives, to say nothing of patients, demand that not too much precious time is spent trying to sort it out.

Stories told of each partner trying to protect the other can seem like an impossible situation that must be put right as soon as possible. I'm not so sure. Certainly not always. After all, for each it can be a matter of satisfaction and self-respect to feel that they are protecting the other. It may seem rather untidy but 'beware the vice of tidymindedness'.

Grief: before death and after death

Grief does not always wait for death. 'I miss her', said a man about his wife with Alzheimer's disease, when she was still living with him. Said another, also coping with a wife whose intellect and memory had deteriorated sharply: 'It's like looking after someone else's wife.' Personality change may also occur with brain tumours. The person we knew and loved has gone. 'There's just nothing there any more', said a wife about her husband.

Quite apart from any personality change or brain failure of this kind, a sense of loss and grief may begin before death occurs. But the extent to which it does is very variable. It seems more likely to happen in a terminal illness lasting a few months than in one lasting either years or weeks. Some people say that they did almost all their grieving before the person died. With the same length of illness another will say they didn't grieve at all until the patient had died – and sometimes not for weeks afterwards. It must depend partly on whether a relative clings to hope or abandons it. And here, as with so many emotions, there are likely to be fluctuations. Days of hope and days of despair. Grief on some days. On others a refusal to give up.

For a few hours and days *before* death – and also during the first few hours and days *after* death – relatives are often more numb than distressed. Remember that some will remain apparently serene and matter-of-fact, though their heart may be breaking. Whether before or after death, never judge the degree of distress by the presence or absence of tears. There are also cultural differences. Loud weeping (by men as well as women) of the type described in the Bible occurs as a normal acute grief reaction in some cultures, but not in others. Differences in different cultures may also be less real than they first appear. For example, it may be that men in our culture are privately just as likely to weep as women, but that this is thought to be embarrassing and unmanly and is therefore hidden.

After death it will seem natural and inevitable to many people that doctors and nurses working in hospital – and perhaps even in primary care – will need to leave it mainly to others to comfort the bereaved. But many in primary care consider this part of their job. A friend in general practice has always made a point of taking the death certificate to the home, rather than asking the family to collect it from the surgery. This serves not only as an expression of respect and concern, it also gives an opportunity to tackle misconceptions or needless remorse. Then another visit about two weeks later – to check that all is as well as can be expected, and perhaps to advise about problems that are only now becoming apparent, for example financial anxieties.

And there are bound to be at least some *hospital* staff, who having developed a warm and affectionate relationship with one or more members of a family during a terminal illness, will not want to forget them completely and will wonder how they are coping with their grief.

Part of a letter from a bereaved relative:

We had some very happy times during the last seven months... we even managed a holiday in London... there was always more laughter than tears.

Though usually discussed separately, there are also these links between terminal illness and grief:

- For some doctors to be natural and friendly with the bereaved is as diffi-cult as being natural and friendly with the dying. So can anything more be done in medical schools to make both easier for them?

- In both situations many relatives are pleased to think that the doctor or nurse may be learning something that will help them to understand other cases better. So whenever this is the case, be sure to tell them.

The reward for good overall care will mean that the family can – at least some-times – see a death, however tragic, as 'a good death'. They can feel pride as well as grief. Their sadness is not soured by doubt, or confusion, or bitterness, or needless suffering.

Though purely anecdotal evidence can be impressive, the value of *special bereavement counselling* should ideally be tested by formal compar-isons of one kind or another – for example between, on the one hand, standard advice and support and, on the other, something much more elabo-rate and time-consuming. Clearly, in both groups all will improve sooner or later. And nearly all will say (if only not to sound ungrateful) that what has been done for them has helped them. But what we need to know, in order to judge priorities correctly, is *how much difference* all the *extra* time spent makes to how the relative feels six months, or a year, or two years later. Parkes says that such studies as there are give conflicting results.[3]

Perhaps surprisingly it has always seemed to me that it's much easier to help the dying than it is to help the mourning. In uncomplicated grief the feel-ing of near helplessness when trying to give comfort can be overwhelming. Whatever we do or say, many are going to have to suffer severely, not just for a few months, but for perhaps two to five years. And there may be times in the first year or two when things seem to be getting worse rather than better.

But if we can't do much about the intense sadness of uncomplicated grief, maybe we can do something about needless or exaggerated guilt, doubts, fears, bitterness or blame. And at least we can shun certain common mistakes that serve only to hurt the bereaved and increase their distress. For example, we can resolve:

- never to try to avoid them without good excuse (one fairly good excuse being that you don't want to hear the same long detailed story more than once or twice – it is up to the bereaved to try not to make this mistake or they will drive people away)

- nearly always to mention, however briefly, the person who has died (the grieving relative then has a choice of either adding to what you have said or changing the subject, but at least you have not behaved as if he or she never existed)

- when possible to mention something once said by the person who has died, or to recall some act of kindness or of courage, perhaps not long before death or perhaps many years ago.

And when you are fairly sure that a relationship (of any kind) was a happy one, why not say, just once, warmly and quietly, 'You must miss him a lot ...' or 'You must miss her very much...'. It seems that in some cultures this sort of comment comes easily and naturally, whereas in others there is often so much embarrassment and fear of triggering emotion that neither this – nor anything like it – is ever said. Which is a pity, because it's not so much the value of what is said, but that if *nothing* of this sort is ever said it's hurtful to the bereaved and isolates them.

Though numbness without any expression of grief is not uncommon at first, if there is still no expression of grief after three weeks or so, this is widely regarded by those with experience as a worrying sign. Worrying in the sense that it suggests that sooner or later there will be a severe grief reaction that may qualify for the term 'pathological' and need psychiatric or other special expertise to treat it.

There may be an element not so much of depression as of a kind of anxiety, a sort of fear, a sinking feeling, a bit like hunger, or convalescence or lack of sleep, yet not quite like any of these. Reassure the bereaved that this is common.

After a long marriage intense feelings may come flooding back of early romantic times together, whether or not the subsequent marriage was happy. And when the marriage has sadly for some years been in a state of conflict, grief may be surprisingly severe. Persistent, too.

For no particular reason some days are likely to be even more painful than others with regard to:

- the intensity of the general heartache and misery

- the ability to cope with normal living

- the feeling of hopelessness about the future.

Perhaps beautiful sunny summer days are worse after an exceptionally happy relationship has been suddenly cut short; with grey days in winter worse if the problem is more one of just being lonely and depressed. And for some people there are surprises, for example suddenly feeling happy for no obvious reason in the middle of intense grief, as described by Kathleen Smith.[4]

> **Relative *(fighting back the tears, a few minutes after her husband had died)*** : *He was no good with the children, doctor. No good at all. But he was a good husband.*

Some things may show little variation for many months or even years. One such is a strange feeling of shock and unreality, as if walking on cotton wool, or being surrounded by a sort of blanket, or living in a twilight, dream-like world, even though able to talk and act in a way that seems fairly normal to others.

Everyone understands how a bereaved person may become tearful when suddenly reminded of something once shared with the person who has died, perhaps a particular piece of music or a favourite place to visit. But more common than many realize are the acute *emotional storms* coming suddenly out of the blue for no particular reason, usually when the bereaved person is alone. Lasting perhaps 5 to 15 minutes, there may be great distress, with not only sobbing and copious weeping, but perhaps even choking and gasping for breath and a feeling of going down and down into an abyss of blackness and despair. After a few months the interval between each attack probably lengthens from a day or two to a week or two, then a month or two, but the victim may be shaken to find that the degree of pain and distress, when it comes, may be just as bad as it ever was. It is as if some chemical slowly accumulates and when it reaches a certain level it triggers an explosive reaction. The rate at which it accumulates slows down, but the reaction when it comes remains as fierce as before.

But remember that, like every other grief reaction, it's not like this for everyone. Other things that may occur include:

- an impression of hearing the person's voice or footstep

- an impression of seeing the person in a crowd of people

- a very intense dream or vision of the person, often never repeated

- a distressing inability to visualize the person's face.

Knowing how much anxiety these things can cause ('am I going mad?' is a not uncommon comment in severe grief reactions) do we warn the bereaved from the start that such things may occur? Or – constantly bearing in mind that there is almost *nothing* that everyone will experience – is it better not to? The problem is that, as previously discussed when warning relatives about the side-effects of treatment, or about what may or may not happen at the very end of life, many people translate a warning that something *could* happen as a warning that it *will*. Then if it doesn't, they may either worry about why it hasn't happened or have less faith in the doctor or other person trying to help them.

Sometimes the bereaved may suffer from such somatic symptoms as chest pain or abdominal pain. Perhaps they identify with the pain experienced by the patient. Perhaps they feel that they, too, may be going to die. Or perhaps this is a somatic symptom of depression.

Especially if death was very sudden and unexpected – or if the victim was still fairly young – there may be a partial refusal to believe that the person has died. One young widow left the door of her apartment unlocked all night for a full six months after her husband's funeral, so worried was she by the thought of him returning only to find himself locked out. It is as if one part of the brain accepts what has happened, but another part refuses to do so.

Example of quite a common kind of what seems at first absurd, irrational guilt after a woman's husband had died:

'I feel guilty because last year I let him go to France alone; he was fine and it all went well, but I shouldn't have let him go alone.'

Is this a case where guilt is 'floating' – as so often happens with anger – and just looking for a target? Or is there more to it?

If only...

It's inevitably quite common to want to put the clock back and to think about how the illness or the death might have been avoided. For example, to dwell on delays over diagnosis – either of the original diagnosis or of a recurrence. Or on a fatal injury of some kind that could so easily have been avoided. Sometimes it's possible to remind these suffering relatives that chance works both ways. There may well have been times in the life of the person who has died when he had narrow escapes, for example by not being in an accident that five minutes later he would have been caught in. And occasionally there may be a case for saying quite bluntly, 'You must try to stop torturing yourself like this, it does no good; life is partly a matter of chance and there's no going back.'

When everyone feels that grieving has gone on long enough, some observers talk as if an effort of will can put a stop to it, forgetting that our intellect can only control our emotions to a very limited extent. However, when after two years or so a bereaved person seems almost not to *want* to stop grieving, it may help to ask gently if the person who has died would want the grieving to go on so long.

As with the dying and their relatives, if we possibly can, we must be glad to see those who are mourning and combine comment on their grief with a little natural, normal talk, say about the weather, or perhaps a bit of gossip that may help to bring them back into the real world.

What seems to be the best proportions of this mix will vary greatly, not only with different people, but also with the same person on different days. Feedback is the answer, and if we are too embarrassed to look the person in the eye, we will not get the feedback and will either fail to cut short what is inappropriate or fail to continue with what is proving helpful.

Other points worth bearing in mind include the following.

- Try never to say (when you have personal experience of a similar loss) 'I know what it's like.' Better to say, 'Nobody else will ever know what you are going through, but perhaps I have a better idea than some.'

- If you didn't know the person well, you can't sincerely say that you will miss him or her, but at least try and say that you expect there are many who will.

- If necessary, go over again the *aim* of what was done both during the terminal illness and when the patient was dying. Try to lay to rest any lingering doubts. They can sour sadness and exacerbate grief.

- If there is family friction over the terms of a will, do what you can to smooth it over, as any ill feeling makes it harder for relatives to share their grief and support each other.

It may help some people, *but not others,* to say:

- 'You are needed and you just have to keep going'

- 'Since one of you had to suffer like this, perhaps you can be glad your wife has been spared this and that it's you who is the one left grieving.'

Some reminders and options

- When considering the relative as victim rather than carer, pay the same close attention to feedback of various kinds – not saying too much or too little, and learning from your mistakes.

- Even in a crisis, when the situation seems truly grim, brief friendly 'irrelevancies' can pay big dividends. Fear is reduced. Trust is increased. And sometimes blessings can still be counted.

- It may be possible to narrow the gap a little between, on the one hand, suffering patients and relatives, and on the other, so-called normal, healthy people their age.

- Concern of the patient for the relative – rather than of the relative for the patient – can be real and moving and needs to be understood and addressed. Relative and patient can each help us to understand the other better.

- Just as we have to try not to make the mistake of avoiding people who are dying – or who are having to watch the dying of someone they love – so we must try not to avoid those who are mourning. In both cases it adds to their distress.

- Don't feel you have done the wrong thing if the mention of a person who has died produces tears. They may be partly tears of appreciation for what you have said – after so many others have avoided any mention of their name.

- If anger and guilt and needless doubts and fears can be eased, a loving relative's grief will still contain much pain, but perhaps there is now more room for proud sorrow and for a feeling that what has happened holds something of beauty as well as of tragedy.

- After perhaps two years or so, though it's probably *not* 'all over' and the bereaved have *not* 'got over it', for most of them the *worst* is over and it's now more, as Longfellow described, 'a feeling of sadness and long-ing, no longer akin to pain, and resembling sorrow only as the mist resembles the rain'.

References

1 Saunders C (1967) St Christopher's Hospice. *British Hospital Journal and Social Services Review.* **77**: 2127–30.

2 Doyle D (1989) Talking to the Dying Patient. In *Talking with Patients – a Basic Clinical Skill* (ed. P R Myerscough). Oxford University Press, Oxford.

3 Parkes C M (1986) *Bereavement,* 2nd edn. Penguin Books, London.

4 Smith K (1979) *Help for the Bereaved.* Duckworth, London.

The relative as parent

Margaret Sparshott

(Note: For the sake of simplicity, in this chapter the baby or child will be referred to as 'he'.)

When we discuss the bringing of bad news to the parents of children, two situations present themselves. In the first case the child may be of an age to understand what is happening and to explain his feelings for himself; he may be of an age to insist on making his own decisions. In the second, the non-verbal child depends on his caregivers, whether parents, doctors, or nurses, to understand his needs and make decisions concerning his future; all responsibility lies with the caregiver.

Each of these situations requires a different approach. The chronically ill child able to communicate verbally may well feel competent to take part in discussions concerning his future, and indeed should be encouraged to do so. But since he is still a child, the parents, who have ultimate responsibility for his well-being, cannot be excluded from the decision making. The doctor therefore engages in a three-cornered discussion with parents and child, and it is important that this discussion takes place in an ambience of mutual understanding.

The baby, on the other hand, is unable to express himself in words. He can indicate his feelings by his behaviour, and experienced caregivers learn to read his signals.[1] Even the very preterm infant can demonstrate distress or well-being, and parents can be helped to understand his ways of communicating.[2] Parents, constantly observing their preterm infant, frequently become sensitive to his needs. But the baby can take part in no discussions, so particularly here an atmosphere of mutual trust must be established if parents are to believe that all is done to keep their baby comfortable, no matter how ill he is.

Pain

The idea that a child may be in pain is very shocking; this is why the first reaction of adults is to deny that pain exists.[3] Sometimes the presence of pain in a child is detected with more sensitivity by the parents than by professional caregivers; doctors and nurses ignore the opinion of parents at their peril. Frequently, however, parents seem unable to perceive their child's pain and can even go so far as to discontinue analgesia on their own initiative. This may be through fear of the child becoming addicted to the drug, or it may be that to acknowledge his suffering means accepting the child is experiencing something that the parents can neither share nor control. In an interview with the doctor the child sometimes admits to extremities of pain he has not mentioned to his parents – maybe to protect them or maybe through fear of not being believed. In these cases it is better for the parents to share in any discussion on pain control, in order that all their fears may be brought into the open. It is much easier to discuss the future of severely ill children if their present suffering is alleviated, so that parents do not have the added burden of this particular anxiety.

Grief

The parents of the dying child need to pass through the process of mourning before they can come to terms with their loss; this process will vary with individual parents and may well be prolonged. Neighbours and friends may fail to understand the profundity of such grief, since the child has had so little time to establish himself in the family. Grieving for the dying child is intensified because of the sense of futility that accompanies it. It is 'against the natural order of things' – life is ending before it has begun. The baby is a symbol of creativity, the child a symbol of potential growth.[4] The parents of the dying child lose not only their present, but their future as well.

In her book *On the Death of a Child*,[4] Celia Hindmarch discusses the breaking of bad news under five headings: 'Why', 'When', 'Who', 'Where' and 'How'. Let us examine ways to break bad news using these headings, but adding another one: 'What next?'.

Why has the situation arisen?

What has happened to the child which makes it necessary for the present discussion to take place? This calls for an explanation from the doctor. In many cases the parents will already be aware of the seriousness of the child's condition – or should be so, if they have been kept properly informed. It will cause considerable heartache and resentment if the parents find that examinations and decisions for treatment have been made without their knowledge. In the case of the critically ill child the breaking of bad news will come as a culmination of events; even so the shock will be great, and the truth is likely to be resisted.

Parents of critically ill children often cope with disbelief by 'playing off' members of the caregiving staff against each other; they seek answers from everyone. This makes it particularly important that the parents should be fully informed of all that is taking place, although it can be tempting, when diagnoses are uncertain, to withhold information until the results of tests are known. It causes resentment in the nursing team if they feel they are forced into deceiving the parents, who in any case may well discover the truth by other means and will consequently lose confidence in the medical staff.

The distress of the parents of the handicapped or preterm infant is nearly always complicated by feelings of guilt. 'Why me?', asks the mother of the sick baby, and she answers herself, 'It must be something I have done'. The mother mourns the beautiful baby of her dreams and has feelings of ambivalence towards the (to her) 'monstrous' being to which she has given birth. Fathers too may feel that it is inadequacy on their part that is to blame. Guilt of this nature is very hard to eradicate; it is important that a trusting relationship between parents and doctors is established from the beginning if future problems are to be addressed in an atmosphere of mutual confidence.[5]

The parents of the handicapped child not only grieve for the normal child they have lost, but must come to terms with an uncertain future. They seem to endure an 'open-ended' grief, since their handicapped child reminds them constantly of the baby they never had.[6] It may take several meetings before parents finally grasp the truth, and they will need time to mourn the perfect baby of their hopes and establish a relationship with the 'real' baby before they can contemplate the years of continuing care that lie ahead. They are naturally anxious to know whether such a thing is likely to happen again, and it is important that they are kept informed of the results of chromosomal and genetic tests. Initially, anger and disbelief are an important part of the grieving process and must be accepted with great patience.

When should bad news be given?

The answer to this question depends on the circumstances described on the previous pages. Generally the passing on of bad news should take place without delay and as soon as those who are most concerned can be gathered together. Bad news must sometimes inevitably be given over the telephone, but this must always be succeeded by a personal interview. If the breaking of bad news must be followed by vital decisions on treatment, time should be given to the parents for them to assimilate the problem and discuss it between themselves in private. Decisions made at times of critical illness must be endured for the rest of the parents' lives, so they should not be made to feel that they have been hurried into making a decision they may later regret.

In the case of children on life support machines it sometimes happens that parents disagree with each other. They will frequently resolve their differences if they are given time and not subjected to pressure.

Who should give the news, and to whom?

Bad news should be given by someone who knows the parents well and has established a good relationship with them. This can in some circumstances be the nurse who has been most involved in caring for the child, but as parents usually have many questions to ask and hard decisions to make, the role of messenger is usually taken by a senior doctor.[4] If the bearing of bad news also involves a decision to terminate treatment, research has shown that, while they reserve the right of making the final decision, parents believe that the doctor is the most actively concerned of the medical team.[7]

Who should be present at such an interview? This will depend on the preferences of the parents concerned and the constitution of the family. The family can be considered either as the nuclear family, consisting of parents and siblings, or the extended family, which includes grandparents and other relatives.[8] Those chosen to be present when bad news is given or decisions are made will be different in individual cases. Some young mothers feel the need of the support of their own mothers, especially if their partner is absent. Some would prefer the presence of a close friend, especially if the friend has shared similar experiences. Some partners may deeply resent being absent from consultation, even if they are not the father of the child in question. Whatever the situation, the feelings of the parents must be respected.

The father of a seriously ill child has his own special problems. In the first place, the mother is likely to be completely preoccupied with her sick baby, and he may be left caring for the rest of the family at home, and with all his responsibilities at work. This may lead to feelings of resentment and consequently guilt. Many fathers feel awkward and clumsy with their fragile infants, but research has shown fathers to be as capable and as emotionally responsive as mothers.[9] Fathers who have participated in the care of their preterm infants during their stay in hospital have been shown to have more interaction with them at a later stage. While at first reluctant to touch their babies, their interest can often be engaged through their understanding of the monitoring and life support equipment, which frequently proves daunting to the mothers.[10]

Siblings should not be forgotten in the giving of bad news; they have sometimes been called 'the forgotten mourners'.[4] Parents tend to try to protect brothers and sisters from bad news, but if children feel they have been deceived it can affect all future relationships with their parents. Children too need to grieve and can be deeply disturbed if they feel excluded. They often have feelings of guilt; death appears as a form of magical punishment, for which the child is responsible through his jealousy[11] – he has 'wished his brother away'. This can lead to withdrawal or unruly behaviour, difficult for parents to support at a time of their own distress. Most children cope better with a shared grief, but they may need to escape sometimes in play, with neighbours or other children who are not involved.

Where should the news be given?

Memories are all that remain for the parents of a child who dies. Inevitably, if this takes place in hospital, the passage of the death itself is going to be the most powerful of these memories.[12] Most paediatric units now have rooms where parents of critically ill children can stay, and facilities for them to make tea or coffee and talk in private.

The delivery suite is not the place for the breaking of bad news. The experiences of some mothers whose babies have been taken from them at birth, and who see, without explanation, doctors and nurses struggling to bring them to life, remain with them as a perpetual nightmare. Of course in an emergency the life of the baby comes first, but an opportunity must always be made later for the parents to have the baby to themselves, in a quiet room.

Some paediatric and neonatal intensive care units have a special private room, non-clinical, nicely furnished and comfortable, where doctors may meet with parents, or where families can get together to share their grief. It is important that this room should be quiet and not overlooked. The offer of tea or coffee may seem banal, but is usually accepted with gratitude; and it is also wise to have a large box of paper handkerchiefs to hand.

How should the news be given?

Bad news should be broken using language that is simple and natural.[4] Such news will need to be repeated; it is often useful if the nurse who has shared responsibility for the child with the parents is also present at the interview, as later she will be able to reaffirm what the doctor has said. Partners should be seen together and encouraged to talk to each other. All the information the doctor has should be shared with the parents, even if the final diagnosis is unsure. All possibilities for the future should also be made plain; if the outcome is unknown, the doctor must say so, even if the parents insist on a positive or negative assessment. An uncertain outcome is particularly difficult for parents as they cannot prepare themselves for either eventuality – death or life – but they will not readily forgive being misled.

The handicapped infant

Giving the bad news to the parents of a handicapped child will take time. Parents need to assimilate such news and the doubtful future it brings, and information may well need to be repeated several times before they can come to terms with it. No matter how severe the handicap, it should never be physically concealed from the parents – their imagination is likely to picture something far more horrific than the reality. The baby should be wrapped or dressed, and shown to the parents while the doctor explains the nature of the handicap.[11] If they wish to, they should be encouraged to hold the baby in their arms while the interview takes place. No matter how severe the handicap, the baby should be respected as an individual. He should be referred to by his name and by gender. In many cases the future may not be so bleak, and the news can be presented in as positive a way as is consistent with the truth. The parents should be assured of continuing support, and later on the appropriate support services can be recommended.

The preterm infant

The parents of the preterm or very light birthweight infant have a long, hard row to hoe. They will need all the information available, and this may change frequently as the baby passes through crisis after crisis. Very often these days the outcome for such tiny babies is good, but their fragility makes them vulnerable, and parents should be warned to expect 'two steps forward to one step back'. Once a good relationship is established between the medical and nursing staff and the parents, however, this is likely to be close and rewarding. When the time comes (as it sometimes must) for a decision to withdraw treatment to be made, this close contact makes it both more difficult and easier for such bad news to be given; more difficult, because nurses and doctors become emotionally bound to the infant and his parents, and easier, because through such an attachment an atmosphere of mutual trust has been created.

The critically ill or dying child

Bad news should be given face to face, and it is important to maintain eye-to-eye contact.[4] All parties should be sitting, on the same level and with no impediment between them. Care should be taken that the interview is not interrupted, that no telephones or bleeps are likely to distract the attention of those present. As has already been said, giving bad news takes time, and it is particularly important to *listen* to the parents. At first they may ask many seemingly disconnected questions; in their distress they may say things that seem shocking, but by listening to them the doctor gives them a chance to get rid of some pent-up feelings. It is natural for parents given bad news to cry, but they should not be made to feel that this is expected of them – it may lead to feelings of guilt if they are unable to do so.[12]

No decision as to future withdrawal of treatment should be taken quickly, as parents should be given the chance to change their minds. Parents can be left with regrets if they are not given a chance to reconsider decisions taken in a moment of great anguish of mind.[4] If they are not subjected to pressure, parents can usually see for themselves when it would be cruel to continue a futile struggle.

The parents of a critically ill baby need to feel that he belongs to them; too often there is a sense of rivalry between parents and staff because parents feel that their baby has been taken over by others, whom they see as better equipped to answer his needs.[13] Instead of feeling responsible for their own child, they feel helpless and inadequate. This feeling of alienation can be mitigated if the parents are encouraged to participate in their infant's care and are consulted when changes in treatment are proposed.

Once the decision to discontinue treatment has been reached, all monitoring equipment not essential for the comfort of the baby should be removed and the parents should be given their baby to hold. Provision should be made for the family to be together in private, but with help available if they should need it.

The older child

The question arises of whether the older child should be told that he is dying. This will depend on the individual child. If he appears innocent and happy, there seems little reason to disturb him. In many cases, however, it would seem that it is better that he should be told the truth – in chronic illness he is likely to suspect it anyway. Some chronically ill children feel protective towards their parents and will avoid discussing the subject with them. Children, like adults, are more afraid of dying than of death. In these days, when death by violence is constantly presented on television and video, the dying child believes that this is the norm. Left to himself he may well perceive his coming death as one of bloodshed and agony. He will need to be reassured about this and be told that death is usually peaceful, and that, as Dr Jolly says, 'the individual's influence and memory live on'.[11]

What do we do next?

The death of a child in hospital is not the end of the story. Usually, once the child has died parents cannot wait to return home, but eventually formalities will have to be completed and arrangements made for the child's funeral. Often the parents themselves, once the first shock of grief is over, will think of questions they should have asked about the child's last illness. The doctor who gave the parents the bad news in the first place is often the best person to see them again to answer their questions or to give them any information derived from a post mortem. The doctor will need to allay any anxieties about future pregnancies – but should never say to the parents, immediately after the death of one child, that they can 'always have another'. It is a mistake for parents to rush too quickly into a new pregnancy; enough time should be given to mourn the child that is lost.

Giving the bad news should always be followed by action. The warmth and reassurance generated by a sympathetic interview will soon disappear if the parents subsequently feel abandoned by the hospital staff. Arrangements can be made for the parents to see a bereavement counsellor, who will explain all the procedures they will need to follow. A list of the many support services should be made available to the parents when appropriate, particularly the Stillbirth and Neonatal Death Society in the case of infant death.

It must be remembered that the parents are not the only mourners when a child dies in hospital. In many cases the child will have passed many weeks, even months, in the hospital and will be well known to all the staff. Breaking bad news will also be stressful for the messenger, particularly as death is frequently perceived as failure by the medical profession. It is often difficult for those giving bad news to conceal their own feelings – but perhaps they should not try too hard to do so. Parents often remember with gratitude the grief shown by caregivers. In fact the absence of emotion can be deeply felt. In their book *When a Baby Dies*,[12] Nancy Kohner and Alix Henley quote these words of a mother whose baby daughter had died:

The doctor acted as if this sort of thing happened all the time. We would have found it easier if the staff had shown some emotion... We had always been told she had her own personality, yet no one seemed to notice that she had gone.

But the parents of another baby, who died almost immediately after birth, tell a different story:

The hospital staff made us feel that this was not just a non-event to be forgotten about... Naomi was important. It helped us to know that the staff themselves were moved by our circumstances.

The parents of critically ill children need to be respected – for themselves, for their child and for their suffering; grief at the death of a child may be common to all, but to each mother and father their grief is unique. What better way to show respect for parents than simply to say, 'I'm sorry'? Sometimes even words are unnecessary – a sympathetic touch of the hand will be sufficient. Whatever method is chosen, parents should rest in the belief that the caregiver also cares.

References

1   Sparshott M M (1990) The Human Touch. *Paediatric Nursing.* **2** (5): 8–10.

2   Sparshott M M (1989) *This is Your Baby: how to understand your baby and what to do to help him grow.* Booklet for the parents of preterm babies. Neonatal Intensive Care Unit, Derriford Hospital, Plymouth.

3   Gauvain-Piquard A and Meignier M (1993) *La douleur de l'enfant.* Calmann-Levy, Paris.

4   Hindmarch C (1993) *On the Death of a Child.* Radcliffe Medical Press, Oxford.

5   Sparshott M M (1996) *Pain, Distress and the Newborn Baby.* Blackwell Science, Oxford.

6   Speck P (1978) *Loss and Grief in Medicine.* Baillière Tindall, London.

7   Shoo K L, Penner L, Cox M (1991) Impact of Very Low Birth Weight Infants on the Family and its Relationship to Parental Attitudes. *Paediatrics.* **88** (1): 105–9.

8   Morris M (1994) Neonatal Care Today. In *Neonatal Nursing* (eds D Crawford and M Morris). Chapman & Hall, London.

9   Beail N (1983) The Psychology of Fatherhood. *Bulletin of the British Psychological Society.* **36**: 312–14.

10 Richards M P M (1983) Parent–Child Relationships. In *Parent–Baby Attachment in Premature Infants* (eds J A Davis, M P M Richards and N R C Roberton). Croom Helm, London.

11 Jolly H (1975) *Book of Child Care.* Sphere Books, London.

12 Kohner N and Henley A (1991) *When a Baby Dies.* Pandora Press, London.

13 Bender H and Swan-Parente A (1983) Psychological and Psychotherapeutic Support of Staff and Parents in an Intensive Care Baby Unit. In *Parent–Baby Attachment in Premature Infants* (eds J A Davis, M P M Richards and N R C Roberton). Croom Helm, London.

Terminal illness

When a person is incurable and unlikely to live more than a year or two, at what point – when talking to relatives – are the words 'terminal' and 'dying' appropriate? It depends partly on whether such patients feel ill or well and on how much they can do, but in general my own preference – and I think that of many doctors and nurses – has been to talk of:

- 'terminal' only if it is *unlikely* (though possible) that the patient will live more than two or three *months*

- 'dying' only if it is *unlikely* (though possible) that the patient will live more than two or three *weeks*.

This is because these words are emotionally highly charged. True, they may be used more loosely in the title of books or articles, but when talking to relatives (or hospital staff) in an actual situation such words have side-effects and should be used with care.

This is not intended to suggest stages that the patient necessarily moves through (though many do) but only the most appropriate words to use when talking to relatives or staff. And, of course, we are talking of probabilities, not certainties. Exceptions are frequent and should cause no surprise.

To refer to someone as 'terminal' when he or she is quite likely to live for a year or two – or as 'dying' when quite likely to live for six months – can:

- mislead relatives and their friends and neighbours

- cause excessive pessimism and a needlessly negative attitude

- have a bad effect on the quality of life of both patient and relative.

In terminal illness short-term goals aimed at improving activity and at least some degree of normal living are often still well worth aiming at. Relatives can be truthfully told that the patient may yet manage small – or even not so small – activities that nobody in the family had thought would ever be possible again. But when it looks like only two or three weeks to go and the patient really is dying, it's unlikely that anything of this sort would be appropriate.

The fears of relatives

Various fears at the time of diagnosis have been discussed in Chapter 4. In the terminal care situation, quite apart from causing needless distress, exaggerated fears can paralyse the confidence and efficiency of the lay carer.

There is a particular need to explore any previous encounter with terminal illness. If there has been a traumatic previous experience in other hands, be positive. Make it crystal clear that you are determined to do everything you possibly can to ease any and every kind of distress. And just as for those still praying for cure (Chapter 4) the story of one patient is enough to give a precious crumb of truthful hope, so in terminal care the mention of just one similar patient may be a great help. But saying that quality of life was improved won't cut much ice. A few details of how it was improved for this particular person are essential.

Especially in the late stages of terminal illness it's all too common for relatives to have misconceptions as to exactly what doctors and nurses are trying to achieve. At any one time there should be one or more definite objectives, such as the relief – or the prevention – of particular symptoms. Such goals or objectives need to be communicated in a positive way, not just to patients, but to as many relatives and health workers as possible, so that

---

One of the reasons for always asking about previous experience of terminal illness is so that if a relative says how much she dreads going through it all again, the doctor or nurse can reply, 'I can see how you feel, but what you are describing sounds like a rather different situation – in any case I'm sure we can do better than that, we pride ourselves on doing better than that. I think you will be surprised how much we can do.'

Something *positive* of that sort. So often in units where there is no special interest in terminal care, comments on how much can be done to ease suffering are too negative, with none of the pride that might be expressed by a team engaged, for example, in heart surgery.

everyone knows the plan. At this stage the worst way to give any remedy is to say, 'What else is there? What else can we do?' – *without any clear goal in mind.*

Most relatives are very grateful when suffering is successfully relieved. But some, like some doctors, are curiously uninterested. The hopelessness of the prognosis seems to be all they can think of. After dramatic symptom relief you ask them how the patient is. You may be speaking to a relative, a nurse or a doctor. And instead of replying 'Weaker, but a lot happier and more comfortable', they say, 'Still going down hill, I'm afraid' just as they did before the pain (or vomiting or shortness of breath or whatever) was successfully relieved.

Death and dying

Many patients and relatives accept quite philosophically that sooner or later we must all die. Others find it much harder. 'What will happen?' is a common question. By which many relatives really mean 'How will he die?', but the word die is too hurtful or frightening to utter. Timing can be difficult, but to the astute observer, small clues may suggest that for some relatives it will be best not to wait too long before dealing with such fears. Quite a few seem to imagine that at the moment of death, as at birth, there is likely to be some distress, whereas this is in fact unusual. Choking is especially feared. If it is the patient, rather than the relative, who seems worried about this, the relative may be the best person – after discussion with a doctor or nurse – to see whether such fears can be gently eased (but probably not to forecast dying during sleep, as some patients are more frightened than comforted by this suggestion).

Sudden death

Some of us will die so suddenly and unexpectedly that we will never know what it is either to have a terminal illness or to be dying. Once upon a time this was feared by the faithful because it left no time to repent. These days – though it can sometimes be hard on the family – it seems to be what many people hope for. But a difficult problem is whether – in cases where sudden death is not uncommon – to prepare relatives for it.

Depending on how likely or unlikely it is, and on an assessment of the ability of relatives to cope with, I have usually tended to warn them.

For example, in cases of brain tumour, where a sudden lapse into unconsciousness could mean that there is no chance for a few last words or demonstration of affection. If this happens, relatives may be very grateful that they were warned – and that each time they have left the patient they have realized that they might not see her again.

On the other hand, some doctors have told me that they would never do this. They feel that it adds too much to the strain that relatives are already having to bear. I can see the force of this argument, but I think it's just a matter of assessing whether the relative is a person better warned – or a person better not warned.

Equally, when the situation is one in which sudden death is *unlikely*, should we tell relatives this? I think we should. It can be very reassuring to know that there will almost certainly be at least some hours of warning. But, of course, the danger here (a danger that will be enough to persuade some doctors never to do it) is the occasional case where, after we have said this, sudden death *does* occur and then the relatives may be angry that they were expressly told that this was unlikely. And they will often forget the word unlikely and say that they were assured it wouldn't happen. But I still think that this is a risk worth taking, at least with *some* relatives.

Moral support for relatives in terminal illness

Explanation, efficiency and moral support for the relative will reduce stress, both during the final illness and later during bereavement. One family doctor, Kenneth Lane, even wrote that when a patient is terminally ill, 'the doctor's influence on the nearest relative is what matters most.'[1]

Whether the patient is being cared for by a primary care team, a hospital team or a hospice team, *esprit de corps* and pride in *efficiency* and smooth running should be just as prominent a feature of terminal care as of any other kind of care. Both patient and relative then feel more secure. There is less anxiety, less doubt and confusion. Less failure to anticipate problems. Fewer instructions that are not clear.

There could not be a bigger mistake than to think that at this stage kindness is all that counts. When each member of a team is calm, confident and decisive – not awkward or hesitant – patient and relative share the confidence that they are in the hands of people who are not just kind, but efficient and confident and professional and know what they are doing.

True and sincere *empathy* is also a powerful form of moral support. It helps a relative – coping 24 hours a day with all the problems of terminal care – if she gets the impression that the doctor has at least some understanding of what she is going through. And also if he or she appreciates that, like the rest of us, both terminal patients and the relatives caring for them may sometimes be difficult and irritable.

And remember that what a carer is going through may well be not just physical exhaustion, not just mental irritability and frustration, and not just anticipatory grief, but distress at the sight of a weak and wasted body, perhaps with undignified regression to childhood incontinence, where not so long ago there was a strong and active man, a tower of strength to all who knew him.

So sometimes ask the relative briefly what the patient was like, in health and strength and character:

- just before the present illness

- when much younger.

It's good to find someone, say many relatives, who appreciates what a change there has been. And yet, as an example of the fact that there is nothing, absolutely nothing, that affects everyone the same way, the wife of a dying man once told me that the only way she could carry on was to think of her husband the way he was now. To recall what he had once been was

---

Remember that what patient and relative have experienced in their years together has not become any less interesting merely because the life of one of them is now moving towards its close. In the last century Charles Dodgson (who as 'Lewis Carroll' became world famous for his book *Alice in Wonderland*) wrote to a friend:

These volunteer visitors are rather dreaded in some hospitals, as they cannot rest without knowing every detail of the disease or accident... we want ladies who will cheer them up and brighten their lives a bit – who will read to them from the newspaper, or get them to talk about themselves or their families... more as a sympathetic listener than as a questioner...

(from a letter in a Torquay museum quoted by Dr M G Thorne)

just too painful to bear, and she would have preferred me not to have asked about it.

The weekly visit

When patients are terminally ill at home, a brief *weekly* visit, no more, can make a remarkable difference to the relative as much as to the patient, provided it's warm and friendly, interested in all problems affecting patient or relative, and positive about what might be done to ease each one. One bereaved woman interviewed by Cartwright described how at the start of her husband's terminal illness her family doctor said he was afraid there was nothing more he could do, so she changed to another doctor and his weekly visits made all the difference.[2] 'If you've got some moral support', she said, 'you can carry on' – this comment strongly implying that she benefited from the visits just as much as did the patient.

Similarly, in hospital it can be a big boost for patient and relative if the senior doctor (in addition to his formal ward round when each terminal symptom and its treatment is discussed) can pay an occasional informal visit – no more than once a week or so – preferably without a white coat on. And, rather than avoiding times when visitors are present, taking advantage of the chance to see patient and relative together for a few minutes.

It's remarkable how valuable this is, *even when very brief,* provided the basic FPI formula discussed in Chapter 1 is remembered. That's to say the doctor doesn't just appear in the hospital ward or patient's home looking uncomfortable, as if performing a painful duty. Instead he shows friendly professional interest in the patient and her symptoms – and also exchanges a little normal conversation with both patient and relative.

Looking back

A little reminiscing can help. If patient and relative have been together for many years (whether as a couple or as parent and child) and you have a spare minute, why not ask them about their early days together? Even in a relationship that has often been less than happy this will nearly always open the door to the memory of better times. What was the worst thing that happened to them in those days? Or the best? And if the doctor occasionally shares a little of her own life and her own childhood memories with the dying patient and the relative (not too much, just a little) that, too, can be surprisingly helpful.

Encourage relatives, too, if they are not already doing it, to talk to the patient of the old days, of parents or grandparents, of family holidays and so on. This is often especially welcome to very elderly people, who often remember their childhood better than their middle life. Such talk seems to have a certain healing effect, especially when shared, provided the memories are reasonably happy ones (or perhaps dramatic and frightening, but with a happy ending).

It's easier to die if you feel that you have led a reasonably worthwhile life. So a doctor can urge relatives to remind patients what they have accomplished and how much they have helped others. This must be sincere and not overdone or done too obviously. But far too often it's not done at all. Don't forget that everyone has achieved something or helped somebody at some time. The self-esteem of terminal patients needs to be boosted by taking every sensible opportunity to remind them of this.

> Unless very weak and ill, everyone likes to feel that he or she is still needed as well as loved – is still able to be useful in some small way. It can be demoralizing for a patient going home from hospital to continue terminal care at home to find that all his normal duties have been taken from him while he has been away. It's worth giving relatives positive advice on this subject. Otherwise, often purely out of misplaced love and kindness, they may make this mistake.

Such talk may also help the more difficult problems of regrets and guilt. Some regrets may seem inevitable – about how things might have worked out differently, how various mistakes were made, or about unfinished business of one sort or another, perhaps some ambition or project that will now never be fulfilled. But the happiest people are probably those who don't believe in regretting anything. A relative can encourage this feeling – the feeling that regrets are pointless.

It's not so easy to help if the problem is not just a simple regret, but a serious gnawing sense of guilt, perhaps associated with past unfaithfulness, deception, disloyalty or betrayal. But something, though maybe not much, can still be done, often with the help of a hospital chaplain (or other spiritual adviser) or psychologist.

Finally, some relatives are puzzled and surprised when, whether in hospital or at home, they find that most of the patient's conversation is as if he is neither terminal nor dying. Ill, maybe, but not dying. The doctor may need to explain to a relative who has not previously experienced it that this is entirely normal and healthy – so long as both doctor and relative are ready and willing to switch to serious talk if at any time the patient seems to want it – before returning to something more cheerful.

Sometimes a patient will be planning his funeral one day (because he fully accepts that he *may* be going to die soon) and a possible overseas holiday the next. Why is this so puzzling and disturbing to some medical and nursing staff? After all, there is a chance that the holiday could occur. A small chance maybe, but certainly not as small as the chance of a big win in a lottery. So what's the harm in planning for it? Many of us would be the same.

To some people terminal patients are not even supposed to have a point of view about anything. Or a sense of humour. Or be experts of any kind, still able to give advice.

Urge relatives (or learn from their example) to continue for as long as possible asking patients for their opinion, even if it's only about very simple matters.

Using the telephone

As discussed in Chapter 2, the 'phone is probably not used enough. It might seem too impersonal a way of communicating in a sad or serious situation. For many years I assumed so. But, provided it contains (which it can do in just two or three minutes) the three vital FPI ingredients (friendly, professional and interested), it may provide powerful moral support in terminal illness. Try it. Then obtain some reliable feedback.

For example, if on the day that patient and relative are expecting a weekly visit, the doctor feels that he can't fit it into his priorities, a 'phone call instead of the visit can make a big difference. Not just a second hand message from a secretary, but a few words from the doctor, including agreement as to whether or not another week can be allowed to go by before the next visit.

This applies just as much to a consultant 'phoning a hospital ward or nursing home as to a family doctor 'phoning the patient's home. But there must be sincere interest – however brief – in the response to treatment and the progress of physical symptoms, mental symptoms, sleep, eating, bowel function and so on.

And never forget that even with very ill patients, it's often possible for at least part of the 'phone conversation to be *directly to patients* rather than just to relatives or nurses. Why not ask to speak to them? When at home, cordless and mobile 'phones now allow even very weak and ill patients to talk to their doctor. If we fail to take advantage of this, it's probably partly due to failing to put ourselves in the patient's place, and partly to the same kind of awkwardness that makes us ask the person accompanying a disabled friend or relative such questions as the classic mistake 'Does he take sugar?' – instead of asking the person directly.

Visitors

- Relatives should be encouraged to arrange for the right kind of visitor to call. The sort needed is one who is happy to talk to fellow human beings, whether or not they are terminally ill, or badly scarred, or severely disabled. Such things are no problem at all to some people but others seem to find them a barrier to natural conversation and good fellowship.

- Visitors will often need to be told not to stay too long. Even a quarter of an hour may be too much, unless the visitor is close enough to the patient and has enough strength of character to sit quietly, neither talking nor listening.

- There is a lot to be said for one person in the family arranging and booking all visits. There is then less risk of days when nobody comes. Or of times when someone makes a special journey, only to find someone else already there.

Outings

The quality of life for both terminal patient and relative can benefit from an occasional outing in a car, perhaps a brief escape to some favourite beauty spot. Maybe a friend or neighbour or local charity can help. The doctor who encourages this – or merely approves – has to accept a risk that, if the patient is taken ill, he may be blamed. Sadly another factor is that some doctors – and some relatives and neighbours – seem to feel quite uncomfortable at the thought of terminal patients doing the same things as people do when they are well.

A young woman who was very weak and wasted, with not long to live, wanted to go to a friend's wedding. For several reasons her mother was strongly against it and asked the doctor – as relatives often do – to tell her daughter that it was totally out of the question. But later, after the wedding, she said how glad she was that she had been persuaded by the doctor to approve. The key feature here was the determination and personality of the patient, whom the doctor had come to know well. For another patient in the same condition the advice might have been quite different.

Prognostic skill counts here. For example, a family holiday may give much pleasure to terminal patients and good memories for their relatives, but must not be left too late.

Friction and reconciliation

To what extent should the doctor or nurse become involved if family friction develops, perhaps financial, perhaps based on old quarrels? Can reconciliations be achieved? That this can sometimes be done is one of the silver linings in a black cloud, one of the reasons why relatives may be glad that the final illness lasted long enough to heal some old wounds.

St Christopher's Hospice, London, has taught us how much can be done in this way, at least in a hospice, where there is more time for it than in a hospital ward.

Where is the patient to go? – hospital? hospice? or stay at home?

Although Hinton's study of 102 dying patients[3] found that physical distress persisted in 57% of patients with heart or kidney disease, compared with only 26% of those dying of cancer, both the public and the health professions seem reluctant to accept this. Everyone thinks of hospices mainly for cancer of one sort or another, and not for, say, a failing heart, liver, kidney, brain or lungs.

Contrary to what some hospital doctors and some relatives fear, good friendly care and attention surrounded by the dying may be a lot less depressing than a poor standard of care in a hospital ward where death is

Terminal patient: *Quite honestly I'd much rather not go home at week-ends, but my wife is so keen that I should, I haven't the heart to tell her how I really feel. Could you tell her I'm not fit enough?*

Patient's wife *(later the same day, to the same doctor)*: *Don't tell him I said so, but please don't send my husband home for weekends; I just can't cope. Couldn't you just tell him he is not fit enough?*

much less common, but where nobody seems interested in either the patient or her problems.

It's sometimes thought that transfer to a hospice is needed for special-ized care, when really what is lacking is basic friendly professional interest. In terms of priorities it's only a minority of terminal or dying patients who badly need either special physical skills or time-consuming listening or coun-selling.

Questionnaires asking people where they would like to die seem to me to be of doubtful value. Most will say 'at home' for ill-thought-out and purely sentimental reasons. Or even, as in so many questionnaires on so many sub-jects (medical or non-medical), because they feel that this is the reply that will look best and the one that they are expected to give. We have all done this when completing questionnaires.

The relationship between the patient and the relative may be crucial. When patients prefer to be in hospital or hospice, rather than nursed in their own home, this may sometimes be part of many years of dislike of any phys-ical or sexual intimacy with their partner. With other couples it may be exactly the opposite. Their main reason for wanting to stay at home together, if at all possible, is to preserve a warm physical relationship to the very end. Another reason for a relative (and perhaps a patient, for the family's sake) *not* wanting terminal care to be at home may be financial – perhaps a daugh-ter will have to give up her job if she is to care for her father or mother at home. Most questionnaires will not reveal either of these factors.

Where dying patients want to be – and where their relatives want them to be – will also depend on the answers to such questions as these:

- will the patient feel *safer* and more relaxed in hospital or hospice, rather than at home, knowing that skilled help will be immediately available in case of sudden distress of any kind?

- who is available at home to do the caring? What is their age? How fit are they? Will the patient be constantly distressed to see what a strain it is for them?

- is it a happy home? Will there be small children, teenagers or pet animals in the house? If so, will they be a help or a hindrance or a bit of both?

- is there a pleasant view out of the window? As Florence Nightingale put it:[4]

  They should be able, without raising themselves or turning in bed, to see out of a window from their beds. To see sky and sunlight at least, if you can show them nothing else. You should therefore look to the position of the beds... if they can see out of two windows instead of one, so much the better.

- how effective and how good at keeping up the morale of patient and relative will be a) the hospital ward the patient could go to, b) the GP and the rest of the primary care team, if the patient stays at home?

- is there a particular hospital ward or hospice (or Marie Curie Centre, or Sue Ryder Home, or nursing home) where the patient will feel safe and is already known to the staff? If so, how easy will travelling be for the relative when visiting?

- is the patient the sort of person who will not mind sharing a room or ward with other patients? Who perhaps even *prefers* to be where there is plenty going on, more to watch and wonder about, more drama, more people to talk to, and *less* – rather than more – peace and quiet? Or is maximum quiet and privacy very important?

When caring at home becomes hard to sustain

It is especially sad when patient and carer become irritable with each other, perhaps because both lack sleep and both are being ground down by a humiliating struggle against bowel and bladder problems, to say nothing of the appalling difficulty for the elderly relative of trying to turn, let alone lift, a weak and heavy patient, even when given special instruction on the subject by a helpful community nurse or family doctor.

The long hours of darkness are not only a great trial for the patient who cannot sleep, they are sometimes as bad – or worse – for the relative, called to deal with this or that problem all through the night. Mental agitation and confusion is often worse at nights. Coping with it adds to the relative's distress and exhaustion.[5] The secret is to anticipate breakdown before it occurs – family doctors and community nurses are the best judges of when this point is drawing near.

An unwise previous promise by a relative never to agree to someone going into an institution of any kind, but always to keep them at home, can be a problem. A brief visit to a hospital or hospice unit may help, coupled with stressing that what is proposed is only for a *trial period* of say, a few days – coupled with a firm promise to take the patient back home at once if it doesn't work out.

Many patients who at first dread leaving home are later glad they did so. With less irritability and tiredness, there may now be a return to more mutual affection between patient and relative. And never forget that there is no good reason why there should not still be just as good a chance of getting out for a drive in the country, or even a weekend break. Hospices and hospitals are not prisons. Or, if they are, they shouldn't be.

Every opportunity must be taken to stop a carer feeling guilty about handing over the patient in this way. If a relative has done a good job of caring and if you admire her efforts, be sure to tell her so. Explain to her that you have seen many patients far less well looked after. Remind her of the advantages to the *patient*, not just to her, of the move.

A temporary rest for a week or so, while others take over, may also be a great help to some relatives, allowing them to recharge their batteries, so to speak, before returning to the care of the patient. But bear in mind that sometimes after a rest, relatives seem less, rather than more, able to cope: the momentum that kept them going has gone.

How accurate can a prognosis be at this stage?

A way to improve prognostic skills is to make private predictions in a pocket diary. For example, if you think that a terminal patient has about three weeks to live, turn to a date three weeks ahead and write down a quick coded message that means 'Three weeks ago I felt that John Smith would die about now.'

In the final weeks relatives often ask how much longer it will be. A common problem is at what stage a distant relative should be summoned. A son in America, for example. If he comes too soon he may have to go back home and have the expense of returning again for the funeral. Too late and he is upset that his mother died before he could get to the bedside. Forecasting can be difficult, and nobody can get it right every time, but I have often found it useful to say, 'A lot will depend on whether or not...' – and then refer, for example, to the function of heart, liver or kidneys.

This gets away from a straight unconditional prediction, which can so easily be misunderstood or turn out wrong. It also gets away from the idea of the steady unstoppable deterioration sometimes assumed by relatives. In its place it puts something that can still be changed by unpredictable events. This is not the 'cover-up' or 'fudging' it is sometimes supposed to be; it is actually nearer the truth.

I had always thought that the nearer the end the more accurate the prognosis was likely to be, but studies have shown a tendency for survival at the very end of life to be shorter than staff predict.[6,7] Two factors are of crucial prognostic importance (both of them, in my experience, being more helpful than any tests, scans or investigations).

First, when seeing a patient for the first time near the end of life and wishing to assess the prognosis, ask either a relative or one of the nurses concerned, however junior (or even hospital cleaners, some of whom become quite astute in these matters), if they have seen any change over the last week or so. This can be very helpful. 'About the same' sends out a very different message from 'I have seen a big change just in the last few days'.

Great care has to be taken not to miss some treatable complication (for example, internal bleeding) that is the cause of this change. But if there is nothing of this sort, the simple observation of a change in appearance, loss of interest in surroundings and so on, progressing fairly quickly, is likely to be a more reliable indication of a short survival time than any biochemical test.

Second is the Karnofsky index (Karnofsky himself called it the Performance Status). This was originally one of four measures suggested in order to evaluate clinical improvement after cancer had been treated with chemotherapy. It was concerned only with the extent to which normal activities were impaired. His other three measures were subjective improvement (including various aspects of what we now call quality of life), objective improvement and duration of improvement.[8] The index was not intended as a guide to prognosis, but it was later realized that it was in fact very useful in this regard.[7]

When relatives can't face the final hours occurring at home

Some relatives are happy to cope with terminal care, but *not* with the actual dying. They dread this happening in their home. They seem almost super-stitious about it. Perhaps they would not be so reluctant had they not been so shielded from death when they were young.

Some doctors – both GPs and consultants – don't question this and readily agree that an ambulance to take the patient to hospital will be the best thing as soon as death seems imminent. Others feel strongly that this should be avoided if possible. They feel this because of:

- the risk of increased discomfort, disturbance and indignity during trans-port

- the risk of being resuscitated in the ambulance. It may be very difficult for well-trained and dedicated ambulance crews, if someone stops breathing, not to do this – even though most of them would *not* want it done on themselves if they were ever in this situation

- the risk of going to some hospital or hospice where nobody knows the patient; to die (perhaps within 24 hours, among strange faces)

- the risk of relatives feeling guilty throughout their bereavement about having given up caring just before the end. This problem is less common if suitable relatives are given basic instruction about death in the home, what to expect, what to do and especially what *doesn't* need to be done.

'You are looking very smart this morning', I once said to a relative on her way to visit her terminally ill husband, 'Are you going to a wedding? 'No', she said, 'I'm just trying to cheer up my husband…'.

Useful options and reminders

- Discourage relatives from using the words 'terminal' or 'dying' too soon. Keep 'terminal' for a probable outlook of less than two or three months and 'dying' for less than two or three weeks. Otherwise it's likely to have a bad effect on the quality of life of everyone involved.

- Many people assume that kindness and honesty towards patients and relatives are the two things that matter; but FPI – friendly professional interest – together with efficiency, is often what matters most for both groups.

- Relatives may have views, especially with cancer, on whether to go on fighting disease or to concentrate purely on symptom relief (avoiding anything that might merely prolong dying). If they find it difficult to know what they hope for, be understanding. Avoid insisting that they make up their minds one way or the other.

- There will sometimes be stress and friction within a family, because one relative prefers to give up all hope and another to cling to it. Many will be ambivalent about it.

- It's best to concentrate on positive plans with short-term objectives – and it will help patient and relative if this is stressed to both in a suitably confident manner. For example, that currently the main aim is that within a few days the patient should be getting a better night's sleep. And that if one remedy doesn't work, there is always something else that can be tried.

- Whether patients and their relatives prefer the patient to be in hospital, in a hospice or in their own home will depend on various factors, most of which cannot be anticipated until the time arrives. An important factor may be ease of travel for the relative.

- Prognostic skills in terminal care may be important, for example if a close relative is overseas. They can be improved if the doctor sometimes makes a quick coded private note of his prediction. Then he can see how often he gets it more or less right.

- When death seems likely within 24 hours, inappropriate emergency transfer – from home to a hospital or a hospice – can often be avoided if caring relatives are given the confidence to cope at home.

References

1   Lane K (1969) *The Longest Art*. George Allen and Unwin, London.

2   Cartwright A, Hockley L, Anderson J L (1973) *Life before Death*. Routledge & Kegan Paul, London.

3   Hinton J (1963) Physical and Mental Distress in the Dying. *Quarterly Journal of Medicine.* **32**: 1–21.

4. Nightingale F (reprinted 1960) *Notes on Nursing.* Dover Publications, New York.

5   Lugton J (1987) *Communicating with Dying People and Their Relatives.* Austen Cornish, London.

6   Parkes C M (1972) Accuracy of Predictions of Survival in Later Stages of Cancer. *BMJ.* **2**: 29–31.

7   Evans C and McCarthy M (1985) Prognostic Uncertainty in Terminal Care: Can the Karnofsky Index Help? *Lancet.* **1**: 1204–6.

8   Karnofsky D A and Burchenal J H (1949) The Clinical Evaluation of Chemotherapeutic Agents in Cancer. In *Evaluation of Chemotherapeutic Agents in Cancer* (ed. C M Macleod). Columbia University Press, New York.

Journey's end

It's important that interest should not slacken simply because the end of life is approaching. The relative needs to see that the doctor is still concerned and still showing a keen interest a) in the *patient's* current symptoms, discomforts and anxieties, and b) in the *relative's* distress and any new anxieties that he or she may have.

A patient with widespread myeloma bone deposits had severe pain on the slightest movement. He dreaded going for scans or X-rays every time a new pain developed, so it was agreed that there was no more need for this. One day, in spite of this, he went for further X-rays. Why? Because the relatives had been asking if there was not something further that could be done. 'I felt I had to offer the relatives something', said the doctor who ordered them.

Moral: One thing to avoid as much as possible (though these days it's easier said than done) is to order investigations that are not really needed, purely in order to impress patients or relatives that you are still busy doing things. In this man's case it wasn't just a waste of resources; it was cruel. Why couldn't this have been explained to the relatives?

Should children visit at this stage?

Relatives often ask for guidance on this point. One relative may be in favour, another against. Sometimes a patient may feel strongly that she doesn't want children to see her like this. She wants them to have only happy memories of how she was before she was dying. Which is very understandable. But in general, provided any pain is well controlled and the patient's general appearance is not too distressing and her personality is unchanged, I think children should visit, because the most likely thing is that it will be good for the patient and good for the children, and both will be glad they did it.

I have a photograph, taken with the family's permission, to show how death can be as natural in a busy, bustling hospital as in the patient's home or in a hospice. An obviously very weak elderly man, his eyes sunken, his mouth not fully closed (he died next day) is sitting up in bed, holding his wife's hand. There are no tubes or drips or apparatus of any kind to be seen. Seated at the other side of the bed is his granddaughter. And sitting on the bed is his one-year-old great-granddaughter. The scene has peace and dignity.

Home visits, family photos and humour

I learned many years ago, when visiting dying cancer patients in their own homes at the request of the family doctor, that if, when you are ready to leave, relatives ask you to stay for a cup of tea or coffee, *you must stay*. Don't ask me why, but it makes the visit twice as helpful. Subsequent feedback from the family doctor or visiting nurse has made this clear.

Be sure and look around for any family photos. Ask who's who and who resembles who. And when the tea or coffee arrives discuss the *past* of the older members of the family and the *future* of the younger ones. Leave the home wishing you could stay longer to hear more.

I once heard someone else say that she had also learned this lesson, but – after seeing a dying patient in his home – she was offered a cigarette with her cup of tea. She felt she had to take it, then spluttered and coughed and admitted that she had never had one before in her life. The whole family were there and they all had a good laugh. And this really helped everybody, though why humour and absurdity should sometimes be so helpful in a tragic situation, I don't know. I suppose it can produce – how can I put it? – a sense of proportion, a sort of peace and calm, and a reduction in fear and depression. The situation is just as sad as it was before, but somehow less nightmarish, more a part of life.

Too many of those writing in recent years about dying have either never recognized the healing effect of humour (of the right kind, at the right time) – or have been afraid to mention it. Once on such a visit I found no fewer than five friends sitting around the bed of a dying man, drinking and laughing with him. They couldn't meet in the local pub, as was their custom, so they were meeting here. It was an unforgettable sight. Not every dying man has such faithful companions, capable of behaving in such a natural and affectionate way, free from any embarrassment or awkwardness.

Not so attractive, but it had its humorous side, was when a dying woman's daughter arrived at a hospital to see her mother, found her father already at the bedside, saw that he had been drinking heavily, and without the slightest hesitation swore at him, walloped him and sent him packing.

Saying goodbye; lucid intervals

Should the doctor or the relative encourage patients to say goodbye to visiting friends or relatives whom they may not see again? It may help grief to look back on it, but it seems that only a minority can handle it. In any case some patients have not yet completely ruled out the possibility of recovery, in which case they may be upset by talk of this kind. And some have difficulty telling dreams from reality, and may get muddled and say things that don't make much sense, or which upset the person they are talking to.

It may help relatives to stress that many people at this stage of their life – though still capable of polite and normal responses – are liable to be very confused in various ways. They may find it difficult to think straight. This doesn't seem to be too distressing to most patients or most relatives, but some find it very sad and upsetting, especially in a person who 'till now has always had a quick and lively mind.

When there are lucid intervals, as is not uncommon, relatives should be advised to take full advantage of them, as each one may be the last. Nothing is sadder than when a last chance to express gratitude or affection is missed, perhaps giving fresh reasons for feeling guilty. During these lucid periods, occasional flashes of humour are an especial bonus to all who have loved this particular side of a dying person's character.

Is it wise to start advising relatives – *before* the patient has died – about what is to be done after death? Buckman thinks this can sometimes be very helpful. Perhaps this is one of those things that has changed in recent years along with the general tendency to be more open and to spell everything out, but I've always been very wary of it. It can so easily sound callous when a friend is told what the doctor said.

Strive to keep alive?

- Sometimes it's a relief for relatives to be assured – long before the final stages of dying – that the doctor is not striving any more to prolong life or postpone death.

- At other times such a statement would sound wrong to them – as it may to hospital staff. For several reasons, though they may have mixed feelings, neither are yet in any mood to give up in this way.

- Then – it may be only a week later – the picture changes and the balance tips the other way. Though they may well hesitate to put it so bluntly, everyone (doctors, nurses and relatives) now hopes it will soon be over, that life will not just pointlessly drag on. You can see the shift in their view partly by what they *don't* say; they are no longer saying what they were saying before.

Example of quite a common kind of conversation with relative when a patient is dying:

Father of dying young man: *It may seem a terrible thing to say, but quite honestly doctor, I hope it will be over as soon as possible.*

Doctor: *It's not a terrible thing to say; that's how I feel, too.* (And a bond of trust has been established, which would not have been possible had the doctor just looked awkward, or made no comment, or made the relative feel that he shouldn't have said what he did.) *Everything we do now has the sole aim of keeping him as comfortable and as free from suffering as possible – but we can't say exactly how long it will be.*

Now what happens if there is a life-threatening infection of some kind? If antibiotics are given purely in the hope of easing distressing symptoms, this must be explained to the relatives. But if we judge that they are unlikely to do this (and may even make things worse for the patient by producing side-effects) what then?

   Or if fluid intake is inadequate, do we give fluids intravenously?

Often these things are decided more by *where* the patient happens to be (in hospital, in a hospice or in their own home) than by anything else. Intravenous drips are far more likely to be set up and antibiotics given if the patient is in hospital and if other patients are being treated in this way. Sometimes, it seems right to resist this tendency very firmly in the hope of a more old fashioned, natural and peaceful hospital death – avoiding needless prolongation of dying. But it may not always be wise to do so. When the patient is in hospital some relatives and some staff seem to prefer intravenous fluids to be given, even though they would be unlikely to feel like this if the patient were in a hospice or in their own home.

Possible additional reasons for some people feeling like this include the following:

- the relative is still praying for a miracle. Perhaps this feeling comes from a persistent refusal to accept the unthinkable. Or perhaps the doctor has held on for too long to the emphasis on 'serious but *not* hopeless'

- the relative can think only of the 'sanctity of life' and, regardless of other factors, of always trying to preserve it

- the feeling that, whatever may happen elsewhere, a hospital is not the place to 'give up the fight'

- fear of feeling guilty. If asked for their views, relatives may be afraid to agree to the suggestion that life-sustaining treatment should be withheld.

This last reason is especially likely if it is an elderly parent who is dying and relatives look forward to being spared the burden of further care – and perhaps of inheriting some very welcome (or even badly needed) money. If such relatives were ever themselves patients in this situation, they would probably *not* want this effort to prolong their life. On the contrary, they may often have said that they resent doctors 'keeping dying people alive'. But now they fear feeling guilty. So, when asking the view of relatives, this possible – and quite common – reaction needs to be borne in mind.

Finally, if relatives ask why such things (antibiotics, intravenous fluids and so on) are not to be given, or are not already being given, it is unwise to reply merely that you think that this would be futile. Better to say firmly that you feel it would be a mistake and – if this opinion is clearly not going to be trusted or accepted without further elaboration – to explain exactly why.

For example, intravenous fluids may be better avoided:

- because dying patients, who are too ill or too weary to swallow more than a very small amount of liquid, do *not* usually suffer from thirst. Perhaps a dry mouth needing frequent attention, but not thirst

- because needles and tubes may well make the patient not only less comfortable, less able to turn in bed, but also generally less peaceful and more likely to have nightmares. Dozing... dreaming... drifting in and out of reality... how easy it must be for the intravenous drip to become an imagined assault or to give a trapped, pinned-down feeling

- because it will mean an artificial intrusion into a last chance for patient and relative to be physically close

- because it might just prolong dying in an unnatural way.

Many relatives are ambivalent and are not sure what they want. Or they may think one thing one day, another thing the next. Sometimes it seems best to attempt – very gently – to reduce this ambivalence and steer them nearer to a definite stance one way or the other. But often it's better to let it be. Note it. Respect it. It may soon resolve. To suggest to ambivalent relatives that they must make up their mind, one way or the other, may just mean that for them there will be less peace of mind, more stress, more unhappiness and a greater risk of subsequent guilt.

Quite often the best way to handle these dilemmas is for the relatives to be *consulted,* but at the same time *protected* from what can be for them the terrible responsibility of decision making. Wilkes put it like this: 'The aim must be to involve the relatives, without abdication from professional responsibilities'.[1]

Euthanasia, advance directives and the use of morphine

How should the doctor respond if a distraught partner or relative urges not just the avoidance of efforts to prolong dying, but maximum sedation in the interests of ending suffering as soon as possible? This subject, like abortion (an equally difficult but far less complex problem), will no doubt be debated as long as the human race exists. For pragmatists at least, there will never be any easy answers. Meanwhile, note that:

- it's very common for such relatives to feel differently only a day or two later after further efforts to ease suffering

- the more the complexities are looked at, the more most caring pragmatists (and even some who are either for or against as a matter of principle) feel that any change in the law would do more harm than good. This was the final *unanimous* opinion of the House of Lords Medical Ethics Select Committee in 1994.[2]

Many now hope that if people make a 'living will' or 'advance directive' there will be less danger of them being kept alive in a way that they would not have wished. It sounds sensible, but public debate of the subject not only reveals various misconceptions, it also underestimates the complexity and variety of situations than can arise. There is also, in my view, a big danger – with some patients writing such directives and others not doing so – that what we used to call 'overtreating' will get worse, rather than better. Staff will be more concerned than at present that, *without* a very clear and strong direction *not* to treat, they may be accused of not fighting sufficiently for life.

Owing to much public misunderstanding it's especially important to explain to relatives:

- that the aim of escalating the dose of morphine or other opiate is usually not to sedate, but to get symptoms under control and hopefully still have an alert patient

- that morphine can be very useful for symptoms other than pain – this is not well known and, unless it's explained, relatives may be puzzled or suspicious

- that neither addiction, nor the wearing off of the morphine's beneficial effect, are likely to be problems. Again, relatives often need specific assurance about this.

If the position is that the patient could die at any time, there is usually no way of knowing whether or not final efforts to get pain under control have shortened life. Many people suspect that this sort of talk is a cover up for euthanasia, when it's not; it may need explaining to relatives.

Certainly there may be a *possibility* that life will be shortened. But to risk this in order to give a better night's sleep to someone who is dying (perhaps even omitting the usual cautious escalation of dose in the case of a hopeless prognosis and an urgent need to relieve severe pain) is clearly a very different matter from risking death in a young person with, say appendicitis, where a certain amount of pain might be judged preferable to even a very small risk to life. This is just common sense and, contrary to what some believe, is an approach that seems quite acceptable to all the main religions, however strongly they may feel about the sanctity of life.

Explaining what is happening

For some anxious relatives – you need to judge which ones – it may make good sense to think of the body as a machine, some parts working, others

> **Dying man to doctor**: *Thank you for speaking to my wife, she is much happier now that she has met you and understands better what you are trying to do for me.*

not. Perhaps mention the deteriorating function of, say, the heart or kidneys or liver, together with a mention of what such organs *normally do* and are now *failing to do*. This can take away fear. And it's something for the relatives to pass on to enquiring friends and neighbours.

For example, 'The reason your husband is short of breath is that the left lung is out of action – his right lung is OK and his heart is OK – but his left lung is out of action.'

- Note the intentional repetition of the key phrase.

- Note also the mention of parts that are working normally. If a person is dying, this may seem irrelevant and unhelpful, but it is another quick and easy way to take some of the fear out of a situation, some of the hurt out of it, some of the feeling of something horrible or unnatural going on, spreading through all parts of the body.

Some other points that may need discussion with relatives

- It's a terrible thing, when a dying patient is still alert, for him to be left *completely alone* at home, knowing – even for short periods, let alone long ones – that nobody is there to answer a call for help. Every possible effort should be made to prevent this, for example, setting up a rota of volunteer neighbours. There are always those ready to help, if somebody can be found to organize it.

- Some patients would rather have pain than side-effects. It may seem to both professionals and relatives that they are being unreasonable, but if we can neither get rid of the side-effects, nor convince them that the symptoms they *think* are side-effects are not, then we should let the matter drop, remain friendly and uncritical, and *urge relatives to do the same*.

- It may be necessary for a doctor to try and persuade a relative to get some sleep at all costs, aiming to convince them that it is in the patient's best interests that they should do so. For a doctor to *order* this sounds like old-fashioned paternalism, but it sometimes works wonders and is helpful to both patient and relative.

- Dying patients often prefer to eat food that the rest of us would say had been allowed to get cold. Relatives must accept this and not worry about it.

- To be worried when hardly any food is taken is also a natural instinct, but relatives may need to be persuaded that it's not at all helpful to a dying patient with a dry mouth and no appetite to be nagged about it. As already suggested in Chapter 7, explain that the body may have good reasons to 'refuse' more than a small amount.

- Sometimes friends or relatives (not the most loving ones, in my experience) even say, 'It's terrible to see him suffering like this', when there is actually *little or no* sign of any suffering. The patient appears to be dying peacefully. But such relatives have a fixed picture of sad situations of this kind. To them such patients are always suffering, and they will report this to their neighbours regardless of the true position.

- Occasionally the attitude of a relative is even less helpful (*see* Box below) but this is, thankfully, uncommon.

Relative *(the dying patient's brother, a man of about 60, with a history of much ill health, who all staff found strange, bitter and difficult to communicate with)*: *He seems to have great confidence in you all, I don't know why, no doctor or hospital ever did anything for me.*

Later a nurse was present when the following conversation took place, probably the last words spoken by the patient:

Patient *(to his brother two hours before he died)*: *I'm very ill, aren't I?*

Relative: *No, you are not. It's just that the doctors have given you the wrong medicine; I'll speak to them about it.*

Nurse *(to relative out of ear shot of patient)*: *Why did you say that to him? You didn't need to say that. He hasn't been given any wrong medicine.*

Relative: *Oh, I know. But I think that was the best thing to say, don't you?*

'Phoning from the hospital

Whether before or after death, it can mean a lot to the relatives to be able to 'phone friends or family quickly and easily without having to wait for someone else to finish what may be a fairly long call.

- Far more pay 'phones should be provided in hospitals for the use of relatives.

- Some, if not all, should be completely soundproof.

- Some, if not all, should have a chair.

Being present at the moment of death

In hospital, be prepared for some relatives to be very upset if they were not present at the moment of death (even if the patient has been unconscious for some time) and perhaps to feel angry that they were not given better warning. This may be part of a general grief reaction, with 'floating' feelings of guilt and anger seeking for something to focus on. But sometimes it's much more than that, so it's very important to establish, *as far as possible*

A man was dying of cancer and his bedridden 85-year-old mother 'phoned. I told her that he might have only a few days to live. She asked to have a word with him and I took a 'phone to the bed and he just refused to speak to her. I begged him to say a few words, but all he would say – in a voice filled with hatred, anger and bitterness – was 'I've nothing to say to her.' I returned to the 'phone and had no hesitation in telling his mother that he was not well enough to talk to her – a white lie that most people, I think, would feel was right in the circumstances.

In the very same week there was another man dying of lung cancer and I asked his wife if she had let her three adult children know that their father might have only a week or two to live. 'No', she replied with bitter anger, 'and I'm not going to. Why should I bother with them?; they have never bothered with us.' 'But surely,' I said, 'they may feel very upset when they hear that you never gave them a chance to see their father and perhaps say they are sorry.' But it was no good. Nothing would persuade her...

(even with just one relative it can get quite complicated), their wishes in this matter and to record them for all staff to see.

- Do relatives want to be informed immediately, day or night, of any important change, so that they can always feel that 'no news is good news'; or do they go along with the principle that, if there is nothing they can do, there is little point in waking them or worrying them?

- Do they want to be called in the middle of the night if there is a marked deterioration, suggesting that death before morning is quite likely? And if they are called for this reason and decide not to come in, do they want to be woken again, perhaps only an hour later, if the patient dies? Or can this wait 'till 7 am or whatever time they wish?

- Such questions must not be left too late, as the patient may die sooner than expected. Occasional checks and modifications may be needed as new factors come into play.

Spiritual support

Obviously if patient and partner practise a religion – or even if they have not done so for many years – a representative of their religion may give them both great comfort, not only while one of them is dying, but also later in bereavement.

And note that the personality of some hospital chaplains is so warm and friendly that without necessarily mentioning anything spiritual they help anyone they see.

Being given a job to do

It can help many relatives to be given a job to do. Perhaps a simple routine task that will at least make them feel they are helping the doctor or nurse in some way. Perhaps counting and recording the pulse or respiration rate (preferably when the patient is unconscious so cannot be disturbed or worried by it). Or something more time-consuming, such as 'phoning round to try and track down something that the patient fancies or which might make her more comfortable, but which is difficult to obtain.

In hospital some relatives may be more than happy to help nursing staff with some task not directly concerned with the patient they have come to see. There is nothing worse for a relative than to feel, whenever they visit a patient, that they are not only of no help but are also getting in the way.

Prayers, poetry and proverbs

Those not helped by prayer may be helped by well-written prose or poetry, not too modern or recent, and quietly and sincerely spoken. This can comfort both patients and relatives before death, and can sometimes comfort relatives after death. Perhaps it should more often be suggested to relatives that they read aloud a favourite poem or piece of prose – perhaps something known since school days.

In the twentieth century we have rather foolishly tended to mock the nineteenth century for this sort of thing. There are signs of the pendulum swinging back a little. Obviously, feedback is vital. If it's not being appreciated, stop at once. Never go on too long. And if the only effect is for the patient to fall asleep, so much the better.

The same applies to a favourite piece of music, softly played, perhaps the same piece at the same time every day. Any form of daily ritual of this kind can be strangely comforting.

'Patch grief with proverbs', one of Shakespeare's character advises in *Much Ado about Nothing*. For many people, whether believers or not, parts of the Anglican *Book of Common Prayer,* written at the same time as Shakespeare wrote those words, can be especially comforting. Quite apart from the meaning there is music in the words. A gentle rhythm, like the wind in the trees, or waves breaking on a sea shore.

Efficiency and explanation

The need for *efficiency* as well as kindness, already stressed in Chapters 2 and 10, still matters up to the very end. For example, in hospital, though most relatives are very patient, long delays after a promise that something will be immediately attended to can be very upsetting.

A day or two before death – or a few hours before – there is quite often a period of agitation and restlessness, usually followed by peaceful (exhausted?) sleep. Some relatives interpret this kind of agitation as a sort of fight to stave off death, but brain failure seems more likely – the patient dreaming rather than suffering – and it may help to stress this. Do we warn them in advance? As with possible side-effects, possible sudden death and so on, that's the problem. However, especially if dying at home, forewarning relatives about this possibility may greatly reduce distress should it occur with nobody on hand to reassure them.

George Orwell wrote, 'It is a great thing to die in your own bed, though it is better still to die in your boots'. And when discussing hospitals as a place to die (for several weeks in 1929 he had been a patient in an overcrowded hospital ward in Paris) he wrote 'in every hospital death there will be some cruel, squalid detail. Something perhaps too small to be told, but leaving terribly painful memories behind, arising out of the haste, the crowding, the impersonality of the place where every day people are dying among strangers'.

In the final hours or minutes, an explanation of the mechanism and process of dying (or what we know of it, including the physiology of Cheyne–Stokes respiration and the fact that it's very unlikely that the patient is suffering any distress from it) leaves a calmer, more peaceful and better understood memory of how the patient died. This is illustrated by the following extract from a letter.

I want to thank you for... the way in which my father, my brothers and myself were helped to understand my mother's last few hours... the easily understood and calm explanations of the sequence of events very greatly assisted us all on that day.

And during the first months of grief, when every moment of those last few weeks, days or hours is gone over, time and time again, such information means less risk of a distressing memory of being left in the dark, not sure what was going on.

Some other points

Tell friends and relatives that if they feel like holding the dying patient's hand – or embracing or kissing or touching in any way whatever – they must not hesitate to do so. The same thing applies after death. But 'permission' to do it has to be given very carefully if it is not to sound like something that you feel they *ought* to do or have a duty to do. The last thing you want is for any relative to feel pressured into doing something they don't particularly want to do or don't feel right doing. Even sitting at the bedside for more than a couple of minutes is more than some relatives can bear. They should not be made to feel guilty if they don't want to do it. But note that they may feel differently if told that there is no reason whatever why they shouldn't bring a book to read while the patient dreams and dozes.

Warn relatives and staff that sense of hearing is the last to go and that anything said at the bedside, unless the patient is *deeply* unconscious, may be heard.

Do we warn of the hostile look that dying people occasionally appear to give their partner, causing much anguish – especially after a happy marriage? Though it's not common, it's so distressing when it occurs that I've quite often warned relatives of this possibility. Is it old hostilities or jealousies resurfacing? Is it the dying envying the living? Or is it a sign of a failing brain and not to be taken as having any real meaning? Clearly the last of these possibilities is the kindest one to suggest to relatives.

Finally, when death is likely within hours (whether in hospital or at home) it can help relatives if a doctor that they have got to know during a terminal illness briefly examines the patient in an appropriately professional way – and then sits with them at the bedside, perhaps for just one full minute (which can seem a long time), saying nothing and doing nothing except calmly observing the patient, then silently leaving.

How can this help? Surely, especially in hospital, with other patients to attend to it is a waste of a busy doctor's time? Strangely, not so. It need usually be done only once. It's partly a mark of respect. And note that if the doctor is awkward or embarrassed it won't help the relatives so much, but it will still help them.

If a patient is still alive several days after it seemed that the final hours had been reached, one consolation for relatives may be to say to them, 'Your mother is putting up a great fight.' I don't much like the phrase myself, because it seldom fits the reality of the situation, but there's no doubt that it comforts some families.

Journalists seem convinced that their readers can't have too much of it. When the popular labour politician, Emanuel Shinwell, who had a reputation as a great fighter, died at the age of over a hundred, there was a report of how he had chosen to leave hospital, serene and happy to be on his way and to die in his own home. So what did the headline writer put above this story? 'SHINWELL LOSES FIGHT FOR LIFE'.

Viewing the body after death

Most hospices provide a special room for this, mainly for relatives who are not present when the patient dies, but many hospitals unfortunately have no such facility.

A tastefully furnished room is best, with an ordinary bed and bed cover for the patient who has died, *exactly* as would seem pleasant and right for a living patient. A warm carpet and curtains. On the walls the sorts of picture (not too many) that suit all tastes and will not offend or seem out of place to anyone. Peaceful scenery, sunsets, woods or fields, children playing and so on. Nothing abstract. And – sadly for believers – nothing overtly religious, because there are so many relatives now who would find this not only unhelpful, but even a little frightening because of the way such images have been used in 'horror' stories and films.

Nobody need stay any longer than they wish. Refreshment is offered. The room must be reasonably soundproof. And, most importantly in my view, there should be a dimmer switch with a wide range that is demonstrated to all bereaved, so that they can adjust the strength of the light to exactly the level they desire.

Asking permission for a post mortem (autopsy)

Though the frequency of autopsy shows marked variations, there has been a fall in many hospitals to less than a quarter of what it was. This followed many years in which it was a routine request, however certain the diagnosis seemed, because you never knew when you might learn something.

Immediately after a death is a harsh time to ask the bereaved for permission, but there often doesn't seem to be any alternative, since asking *before* death seems even worse – and after death there must be only the briefest delay. It used to be always a doctor who sought permission, but times change and the sensitive approach of the person doing it – and the importance of not keeping relatives waiting – probably matters more than who does it.

For relatives the main problems about an autopsy are likely to be:

- just the thought of it being done (which can naturally be quite upsetting)

- irrational emotions ('Surely she has suffered enough?')

- unpleasant images based on horror stories (scientists probing human bodies)

- religious and cultural objections.

However, many relatives also appreciate that, if there is any possibility of it helping others, it might well be *the wish of the person who has died* for it to be done.

There was a time when it could also be pointed out that the best doctors, like everyone else in society with a special skill, have to be constantly learning from their mistakes, seeing what they missed and looking at how accurate was their diagnosis. Many relatives used to be very understanding and sympathetic when this point was put to them. But sadly in today's litigious atmosphere many doctors would be very reluctant to put it like this.

For most relatives the less detailed discussion there is about this matter the better, but if they look worried and misconceptions seem likely, it may be best to stress that:

- after the internal organs have been examined – and perhaps samples taken – the incision is carefully stitched up, exactly as it would be after a surgical operation in life

- after the post mortem the body looks the same as it did before

- the face is never touched.

Another kind of request, much discussed in recent years, is the request for the donation of organs, for example kidneys (healthy because the victim was fit before being involved, for example, in a road accident). The greatest mistake is to ask for permission before the relatives have fully understood and accepted the diagnosis of brain death. Great sensitivity and tact are needed, but it seems reasonable to ask doubtful relatives what they think the victim's wishes would have been.

Finally, after a death somebody must advise on practical arrangements – the choosing of an undertaker, whether or not there is to be a cremation, the registering of the death, contacting a lawyer, and so on, carefully bearing in mind ethnic customs where relevant.

A few points worth repeating

- At the very end of life it will help if you show that you are still interested in both patients and relatives as people with achievements of one sort or another. And in all current symptoms and problems, new or old, physical or psychological.

- There may need to be some discussion of the sort of mental confusion (often with lucid intervals) that is so common. And perhaps of the likely final process of dying.

- Some sensitive decisions may be unavoidable. What is done or not done – and who is or is not consulted – is usually best decided according to the various features of an actual situation. It's often best to *consult* the relatives, but *not* to ask them to commit themselves to a definite decision.

- Respect for ambivalence is one of the keys to wise communication with relatives both before and after a patient's death.

- With appropriate discussion, most relatives – once pain and other distressing symptoms have as far as possible been relieved – will probably prefer the final hours of dying to be as natural as possible, even in hospital, rather than have an unnatural death with tubes and drips getting in the way of love and physical closeness. But some may not be happy with this.

- Explanation and moral support during the final hours will reduce the stress of the relatives, both at the time and later during bereavement.

- When death occurs, refreshment and a chance to be privately and quietly alone with the person who has died need to be combined with practical advice on what now needs to be done.

References

1 Wilkes E (1989) Ethics in Terminal Care. In *Doctors' Decisions* (ed. G R Dunstan and E A Shinebourne). Oxford University Press, Oxford.

2 House of Lords Select Committee on Medical Ethics (1994) *Report of the Committee*. HMSO, London.

The angry relative

The better the judgement of doctors and the better their communication skills, the fewer angry relatives there will be. But no doctor can avoid it all the time. Is there more anger directed against hospitals and doctors than there was 30 years ago? Though there is no lack of thanks and praise, it seems to be so.

Has there been an increase in mistakes, inefficiencies and delays? Or is it just that patients and relatives are less willing to put up with them without getting angry? How much is due to increased expectations?

Many relatives are remarkably patient and forgiving about delay, inefficiency or worse. It's always best to assume – at least initially – that angry relatives have every right to be angry.

However:

- some relatives (more than there used to be) seem unable to regard misfortune as a normal part of life – they always want to search for someone or something to blame

- even when there is no conscious desire to do this the emotional side of human nature finds merely raging against *fate* rather unsatisfactory, so the anger may be subconsciously projected on to hospitals or doctors

- there may be anger merely because of being given bad news (but this desire to 'kill the messenger' is less likely if the sort of advice given in Chapter 4 is followed)

- anger may be an expression of other emotions, such as guilt, or fear or self-pity, though sometimes the most expert psychologist may be unsure of the underlying cause

- anger may be part of an expression of grief and loss (*before* or *after* death)

- just as doctors and nurses can be idealized, so they can be 'demonized' (Murray Parkes prefers the term 'monsterized'), though this is less likely to happen to nurses than to doctors. Once demonized, *anything* said is judged to be insincere.

Relative: *The surgeon says that the operation he's done for a recurrence gives my wife a small chance of not having any further trouble.* (Then, very angrily) *A small chance? What's that supposed to mean?*

Why the anger? It was an uncommon condition, and the new prognosis couldn't be any more precise than that. Nothing was being concealed. Everyone was doing their best. So the anger was hardly fair, but it had to be forgiven because it had clearly been switched from anger against fate to anger against doctors.

Blaming another doctor

Sometimes a relative tells a doctor that he can never forgive another doctor – for example, for saying that his wife's backache was probably just a sprain when it later turned out to be secondary cancer.

Now comes a dilemma. Such anger can be so unfair to the accused doctor that we feel we have a duty to try and set the record straight, to explain whenever appropriate that this could happen to the most careful and experienced doctor, that in no way was this other doctor necessarily careless or incompetent. But unfortunately:

- if the anger is very strong and fixed, it is unlikely that anything we say will have any effect

- it may well damage our future relationship with this relative, who probably still has some spare anger, which will now be directed against us – for seeming only to want to 'whitewash' and cover up for a fellow doctor.

So, feeling rather ashamed that we have made little or no attempt to rescue the reputation of the other doctor, we take refuge in neither agreeing nor disagreeing with the accusation. Instead we change the subject and talk about something else.

Anger for not being given more information

Lack of information is a more likely target for 'floating' anger than it would have been 30 years ago, because this is the mood of the times and because of constant media campaigns on this theme.

If there were more time, non-essential information of an educational kind could be given more often. There is now a great demand for it. But a busy doctor under pressure can only give what it's important for the relative to know. For example, an intelligent middle-aged woman was angry that, in an emergency when her mother had a stroke and was found to have high blood pressure, she was not given a full account of the nature of high blood pressure and its possible causes.

Along with there being less trust, requests for quite detailed information about technique or dose are now becoming more common.

- Sometimes the information given may not be properly listened to by the patient or relative – nor used for any particular purpose – but merely serves as a symbol of being 'fully informed'.

- At other times details are sought with a view to comparing them with what is claimed by friends to have been done in other (reputedly similar) cases, or with what is written in reference books or lay journals.

From the point of view of consumerism this may seem to make sense, but for various reasons there is a big risk that amateur efforts to make complex comparisons of this kind will lead only to serious misunderstandings and false conclusions.

- Anger with a doctor's assessment may be due to relatives having their own fixed theories as to what the trouble is or what caused it. However much we may disagree, it may be best not to ride roughshod over their views, but to be tactful and take them into consideration.

- Generalized criticism of the whole medical profession – sweeping and not clearly focused – often comes, in my experience, from those who would like to have been doctors. Perhaps regret and envy explains some of their anger.

- Sometimes a relative whom one doctor finds difficult and angry is all sweet reason when talking to another; one doctor being played off against the other.

Anger at the time of diagnosis

Relatives may be angry either about a *delay* in making the correct diagnosis, or about failure to make it at all. As with every other kind of complaint at one end of the spectrum may be clear evidence of neglect or incompetence. At the other end there may not be a shred of good evidence to justify such a charge, the angry relative simply not realizing the difficulties. And between these two extremes there will be many, many grey areas.

As mentioned in Chapter 1, apart from the main diagnosis, there is a sense in which a doctor needs to make a diagnosis in the case of every new symptom. Here a potential source of anger, as discussed in Chapter 7, is if it is ever suggested to the relative of a seriously ill patient that *some* symptoms – for example, pain or shortness of breath – may be at least partly *psychological.*

Before they even have a chance to ask angrily, 'Are you suggesting my wife is *imagining* the pain?', it's best to get in first and explain that this is the very last thing we mean. And then try to get across in one way or another – at least to selected relatives – the important concept of somatization of mental distress, explaining that it's not only headache that can have a purely emotional cause; the same thing can be true of pain and other symptoms in other parts of the body.

Anger about prognosis

There may be anger when the prognosis turns out to have been 'wrong'. The word 'wrong' has to go into quotation marks because it may be that nine out of ten experienced doctors would have said the same thing in the same circumstances and would do so again. The way things turned out was always a *possibility,* but never a *probability.* And this remains just as true as it was before.

- In spite of all our efforts to explain this, relatives may not realize the full range of unpredictable individual variation and the extent to which it's only probabilities and possibilities that can be offered.

- In the course of an illness, both in the short term and in the long term, there may be repeated improvements, setbacks, disappointments, doubts and pleasant surprises.

- If anxious relatives keep asking different members of staff for their view of what's going to happen next, it's as certain as night following day that they will get conflicting (or apparently conflicting) opinions.

- When pressed to make a forecast of some kind a doctor's opinion that something *might* happen is far too often quoted by relatives as a statement that it will happen.

To avoid this:

1   First try to establish rapport and trust – and then gently suggest to relatives that they avoid as much as possible requesting opinions from other members of staff.

2   It may be wise, especially with some relatives, to ask whether they have talked with any other member of staff since you last spoke to them, or have asked other staff the same question(s).

3   As discussed in previous chapters, when the patient is in hospital and several specialists are involved, it is best that *at any one time* just one should be 'in the driver's seat'. The relative should know who this is. It will not always be feasible to confine communication to this one person, but this should be done as far as possible.

4   Relatives should sometimes be asked, when quoting what they have told to friends or family, to try not to omit words like 'may', 'might' and 'possibly'.

When the prognosis was given was there excessive optimism or excessive pessimism? Some of the advantages and disadvantages of optimism and pessimism have already been discussed in Chapter 5 and elsewhere. Here let me just stress that, like Conan Doyle and John Ryle, but contrary to the views of many doctors, I believe that pessimism is actually *more,* rather than less, likely to arouse anger if it turns out to be wrong.

But everything depends on the quality and sincerity and balance of the optimism. None of us will get it right every time, but when everything goes wrong and optimism is followed only by deterioration and disaster, there may follow not the anger that might well follow insincere, casual or excessive optimism, but a sadness and disappointment that doctor and relative share. Events have dashed the hopes of both of them.

Stranger on a train *(showing intense, bitter, smouldering anger)*:
*They told me that my father could live for two years. Then he died in two
weeks. That's doctors for you.*

Doctor: *Be fair, it's not easy; he didn't say your father* would *live two
years, did he? He wanted you to know that he* could *easily live for two
years. I don't suppose anyone could possibly have known he would die so
soon...* (But my fellow passenger was now looking more hostile than
ever... I'd have done better to have kept my mouth shut.)

Treatment

Cure

With the benefit of hindsight, relatives (especially those of cancer patients)
are sometimes distressed and angry because they feel that the treatment that
failed was needlessly drastic. Little can be done other than to go over again
the ground covered before the treatment was given – the hopes, the fears,
the experience with previous cases; the fact that some outcomes are successful, some are not; the grim outlook if this treatment had *not* been given;
and the evidence (preferably backed by randomized trials) that less drastic
treatments give less chance of success.

It's much less common for relatives to feel that the treatment was not
bold and drastic enough, though this may well be the case. Many people –
perhaps inevitably, if illogically – are more distressed by one death resulting
from attempts to cure than they are by two 'natural' deaths due to treatment
that – in an effort to reduce side-effects – was too timid.

Another occasional cause of anger is after being told that, 'In this situation there isn't really anything you can do to make recurrence less likely.'
How far do we go down the road of inventing things for which there is no
real evidence, as is done so often in alternative medicine, in order to give
patient and relative the feeling of still 'being in control'?

What if something that is remote or unlikely – it may be a complication
of the disease, it may be a side-effect of the treatment – turns out in the event
to be all too real? If it was always recognized as a remote risk, but considered too remote to need routine discussion with every patient and relative,
then, though many are very understanding, some will be angry.

It's occasionally possible to put to such relatives – if they are not too angry – the case for not always adding to stress and anxiety at the start of treatment by listing all the remote risks. Are they really sure that they would always do this if they themselves were doctors? Can they honestly say that they do it now with their own ill friends and relatives (not just some but all of them including the most elderly?)

Symptom relief

When attempts at cure or prolonging life are abandoned, this must be made plain to the relative. From then on every single thing that is done must have a specific goal in terms of a particular kind of symptom relief, or a better quality of life. This must be explained to relatives, if they are not to be needlessly confused or dissatisfied.

The danger is that because the outlook is so bad, nobody is very interested, nobody really listens to either patient or relative and nobody studies the symptoms properly. Or that promises are made to patient or relative and then not kept (partly because purely palliative care is given too low a priority by some doctors and some hospital units).

However, once again, it's also possible that the standard of care is in fact reasonably good, but that relatives have excessive expectations.

Anger about the patient 'being a guinea-pig'

As discussed in Chapter 6, it may have to be explained to anxious relatives as well as to patients that the most reliable way to compare two ways of treating a condition is for patients to be allotted to one or other method according to chance, thus eliminating bias and finishing up with two groups that are the same apart from how they are treated. The history of medicine shows that unless this is done it's very easy to arrive at false conclusions as to which treatment is best – and which is only second best or even doing more harm than good.

For many years it was felt that if both of the treatments being compared were normally regarded as appropriate (that is to say, not experimental or unusual in any way) – and if nobody knew which was the best – *and* if the doctor would be happy for himself or one of his own family to have their treatment randomized in this way, there was no need to discuss the matter with the patient or relatives. The feeling was, that because of the anxiety and confusion that this could cause, it was often more ethical *not* to discuss it.

Now all that is changed. First in the USA and then in Europe it became generally felt (not always sensibly in my view, but we have to accept that the whole culture of society is changing to some extent) that all disadvantages must give way to the one overriding principle of being more open, and that whenever a randomized comparison or study is contemplated (no matter how harmless, no matter how ethical) no patient should be included without special consent, following adequate explanation.

If something goes wrong, or if there are serious adverse effects from the treatment, it's usually illogical to blame the fact that treatment was randomized. Exactly the same thing might have happened had the treatment not been randomized. But the 'guinea-pig' image is a very powerful and emotive one, and it may sometimes be difficult to convince angry relatives of this.

When things go wrong, possibly leading to legal action for negligence

Remember that:

- things can go very wrong without there being any error

- errors do not necessarily constitute negligence

If errors occur it is usually best (preferably after sharing with one or more colleagues what has happened) to give an *immediate* explanation to both patient and relative, perhaps seeing them together, perhaps separately, *making it clear that everyone concerned is deeply upset that such an error should have occurred*. It's *not* true that the medical defence societies advise that nothing should be said before legal advice has been obtained. On the contrary, they advise immediate frankness and open expression of concern for what has happened.

At the same time it's obviously fairer that, as far as possible, nobody (particularly someone who might be regarded as being partly responsible) should attempt to apportion blame at this stage. That will come later after a full enquiry. When things go wrong it's seldom – even when there seems at first to be only one cause or only one person responsible – that there are not one or more contributory causes. For example, there may be a case for saying that there should have been more supervision or more training.

So:

1   describe the error, but try and avoid apportioning blame

2   express an appropriate degree of concern and regret

3   promise a full enquiry.

Fear of litigation is certainly *not* the main reason for advocating the approach to partners and relatives outlined in this book. Nevertheless a warm relationship, coupled with confidence in the doctor's ability, will:

- make anger – whether or not it is justified – less likely (or, if it occurs, less intense)

- make legal action less likely.

Half a century ago it was observed[1] that:

It is easier, often enough to have the patient's confidence, than it may be to gain that of the relatives, of whom there may be several. Perhaps after a consultation all is serene until some neighbour calls to enquire and express dissatisfaction.

Now it is often a distant friend or relative living in another country – perhaps in the USA where litigation is more common than in the UK – who urges suing for negligence.

Legal action may be rationalized and justified by a claim that it is not retribution or compensation that is being sought. On the contrary, say many relatives, their sole desire is that everything possible is done to see that it doesn't happen to someone else.

So every possible effort must be made to convince angry relatives that nobody feels more strongly about this than the medical or nursing staff involved. However, *how* this is said – and the timing of it – can be difficult because with some relatives, especially in the immediate aftermath of a mistake, to stress this point may only increase their anger. Why are extra precautions, they say angrily, only now – when for them it is too late – being put into effect?

Quite apart from these aspects, there seems to be far more demand than there used to be for *exact details* of what happened. To supply this can be difficult and time consuming. Also different members of staff may remember things differently. Some relatives will know from experience in their own life how inevitable this is, but others may become even more angry and suspicious when any discrepancies arise. Somebody must be lying, they say. Well, perhaps they are. But often it's not so. The different versions of what happened may be completely innocent.

An 81-year-old woman falls and fractures her femur. An unexpected finding is secondary cancer (primary unknown) in the bone at the site of the fracture. It is felt that she is well enough to be transferred to a hospital 25 miles away for two days gentle radiotherapy, the aim being a) to relieve pain and b) to help the fracture to heal. But a message is received that the family all agree that they don't want their mother to have this.

With other patients waiting for treatment (and with great pressure on resources) it's tempting just to accept their wishes and to cancel the treatment. On the other hand it seems likely that the family's view – as so often happens – is based on serious misconceptions such as:

- a fear of unpleasant side-effects (the truth being that in this case there are very unlikely to be any)

- a mistaken belief that the advice is just an unthinking reflex medical response to the situation, planned without regard to the patient's age and incurability.

So a special appointment is made, and after a full 20-minute interview with one of her daughters (the doctor answering all her questions and repeatedly stressing that he is only wanting to do what he would want for his own mother in the same position) it is finally agreed that she is transferred.

She seems quite happy with both the journey and the radiotherapy, but next day has a stroke and dies. Four *very angry* relatives (three daughters and a son) then ask to see the doctor in order to tell him that they were right all along. They *'knew'* that something like this would happen if their mother were transferred for radiotherapy.

Was it a mistake to transfer her? With hindsight it was a disaster. Without hindsight it put the interests of the patient firmly before the inexperienced views of the relatives, but was that wise?

What can be done when a relative is angry?

Personally I owe much to those nurses, social workers, doctors and others who have shown me how they coped with angry relatives and how they dealt with situations that would have defeated me. Often the secret of their wisdom, understanding and tact was too subtle to put into words.

Many doctors have experience of being anxious or angry when they themselves have been either patients or relatives. This should help them to be understanding. A fairly recent phrase – at least, recent to those like me with no formal training in psychology – that I find helpful is the concept of 'giving permission' for people to feel angry when misfortune strikes. It may clear the air and help to deflect the anger away from others who don't deserve it.

In the case of angry complaints, always *listen carefully* and in such a way – and with sufficient comment on what you hear – that the angry relatives is satisfied that you really *have* listened. The problem now is not the glazed look of *relatives* not listening properly (as discussed in Chapters 1 and 4) but the glazed look on the face of *doctors,* nurses or administrators that convinces angry relatives that *they* are now the ones who are not really listening. This can only increase the relative's anger.

When there is *extreme* anger and bitterness all the sympathy and understanding in the world will be of no avail. Any attempt, no matter how sincere, either to claim empathy or to suggest that it could have been worse will be rejected as insincere and hypocritical.

To try to explain that guilt and other emotions can easily be transferred into anger is even more likely to increase, rather than decrease, their anger. In general be sensitive and understanding about this probability or possibility, but do *not* discuss it or confront a patient or relative with it. Angry people are in no mood to listen to lectures (unless perhaps done *very* cautiously and tactfully at a later stage with those relative whose anger has cooled and who seem as if they might be able to accept it).

Frequently, even when fairly certain that criticism is undeserved, it may be best not to argue. Doctors must try not to mind if a distressed relative sometimes seems illogical, ambivalent and unreasonable. Instead they must be very forgiving and sometimes be prepared to accept the role of scapegoat without complaint.

At the same time, very occasionally, a fairly sharp retort – from a caring and busy doctor to a relative who is being very unreasonable – can pay off, as shown by a subsequent apology from the relative to the doctor concerned.

> **Sometimes relatives who are critical of _another_ doctor – one who has perhaps clearly made a poor job of communicating with them and with others – should be reminded that doctors are only human; that few, if any, can be good in _every_ way; and that a doctor who is known to be a poor communicator may, for example, be an exceptionally astute diagnostician and thus save a patient's life in a situation where another doctor, who is a better communicator, might fail.**

Finally, though the main concern of doctors should always be for patients and their relatives rather than for staff, some thought needs to be given to the caring young doctor or nurse who may be deeply upset by a complaint, and who may be tormented by guilty feelings, which most people who hear the facts would feel were largely – even entirely – unnecessary. Such a person needs support and reassurance.

The relative who is angry with the patient

When the relative is angry with the _patient_ this may be either at diagnosis, during the burden of caring or as part of a grief reaction after a patient has died.

- It may be that the patient did not seem to make any attempt to modify his life-style in the way his partner begged him to (for example, making no serious attempt to give up smoking, then later contracting lung cancer or another smoking-related disease).

- The patient may have refused medical advice (as mentioned in Chapters 6 and 11), and this may make the relative angry.

- The anger may be based on jealousy or on something difficult to forgive, perhaps dating from many years ago.

- Sometimes, in _bereavement,_ there may be irrational anger against the person who has died for dying and abandoning the relative. This, of course, may be followed by guilt at having such feelings – then yet more tension and anger. It may be enough to assure the relative that such feelings are not uncommon and will pass, but sometimes expert psychiatric help may be needed.

Guilt dressed up as anger is especially common when very *elderly* patients have been living on their own and a son or daughter shows anger and irritation, rationalizing this in various ways, for example angrily criticizing the old person for insisting on living alone, when it might be more reasonable to admire their courage for wishing to remain independent for as long as possible.

Guilt in such cases can either be about having not been sufficiently considerate in various ways, or more specifically about not wishing to have their elderly relative live with them. Perhaps there is added guilt and anger at the thought of what friends and neighbours may be saying.

Finally, not only can some elderly patients be difficult, critical and never satisfied, but sometimes, even more sadly, the sheer goodness and patience of an elderly relative ('Be sure to let me know if I'm being a nuisance, won't you?') can trigger intense irritation, especially when the carer can seldom get away from it. And in this case, of course, guilt will follow, further adding to stress.

To sum up:

- There is never an unlimited amount of time. Priorities have to be set. But there will be fewer angry relatives if students and trainees show friendly professional interest at all times – to relatives as well as to patients – perhaps they can find time to pick out, from the suggestion in this book, the options best suited not only to the relative they are speaking to, but also to their own personality.

- Mistakes and misunderstandings occur in all human affairs, but with illness or injury they will be especially resented. They should usually be immediately reported to patients and relatives and appropriate concern expressed, but as far as possible avoiding apportioning blame until the completion of a full enquiry.

- The reasons people give for their anger are not always the real ones. Misfortune may create a 'floating' anger that is looking for a target.

- There is probably nothing that can be said to an intensely angry relative that will immediately reduce their anger. All that can be done at this stage is to avoid saying or doing anything that will increase it.

- In emotional, life-and-death situations, just as some doctors may be given more credit than they deserve, so others may be quite unjustly denigrated.

- Relatives may also become angry with the *patient* (often from guilt, which needs to be understood) or with other relatives.

The angry parent *(by Margaret Sparshott)*

Rage, rage against the dying of the light

(Dylan Thomas)

Anger is part of the process of mourning. It can be directed against the sick or dying person for his desertion of the bereaved, at the medical staff who are perceived as 'responsible' for the situation, and at the angry person himself, who has feelings of guilt.[2] Anger is often associated with fear and is therefore useful in that it compels the person to defend himself; but of course if he does not know what to fight, anger is linked to frustration.

being angry at the situation, recognising it as something rotten, unfair, and totally undeserved, shouting about it, denouncing it, crying over it, permits us to discharge the anger which is a part of being hurt, without making it harder for us to be helped.

(Harold Kushner[3])

Let us look at an illustration of this.

> While I was a nurse on a neonatal unit in Geneva, I was confronted by the father of a very sick baby, wild with anger at the circumstances that had disrupted the routine of his life. He searched for the most insulting thing he could think of that would hurt me, and 'vous êtes un cheval!' he said. Not wanting to antagonize him further, I made no reply, but carried on with my work – in any case, what was there to say? I was intensifying the distress of his sick child even further by inserting a cannula; the father saw his child crying and could do nothing to help him. Later he apologized, very embarrassed; it turned out there were other troubles in his life, as if anxiety for the baby and having his wife devote her whole time to the hospital were not enough. As it happened, to be called 'un cheval' was no great insult to an Englishwoman who loves horses; if he had called me 'une vache', I might have been more offended – but even in his fury he would not have gone that far!

This father was filled with anger – but at what? He knew I was doing the best I could for his baby, that I had not been the cause of the illness, that I was no more than a cog in the wheel of the traumatic but therapeutic structure employed to keep fragile babies alive. He was angry at a vague, amorphous 'something' that threatened the well-being of his family, but which it was impossible directly to attack. I was the nearest object, so he attacked me.

Anger at the death of a baby or young child is usually aimed at the *cruelty* of the situation and the *impotence* of the parents in the face of it. As mentioned in Chapter 8 a fury of frustration is aroused at the waste of a life that has hardly begun: 'It seems senseless, beyond understanding, a complete reversal of all that has been expected and hoped for'.[4] Anger and bewilderment combine in hatred – of themselves, of other 'successful' parents, of doctors and nurses, of a God who allows such things to happen. It is a sad fact that faith in God often fails at such times; one father described how he 'wept and screamed in anger with God after his son died in spite of all his prayers for his recovery'.[5] Eventually religious faith (whatever the religion) may be of help to a believer, as the bereaved parents come to terms with death.

Since the parents of babies and young children are often young themselves, the loss of their child may be their first close experience with death, and fear of death adds to their shock and bewilderment. Perhaps saddest of all, young mothers frequently develop a self-loathing, a detestation of the body which has so failed them: 'I hated my breasts for producing milk where there was no baby to feed'. Parents sometimes blame each other for their loss – parents of handicapped children frequently blame each other for the abnormality – and it takes great patience and a strong mutual bond to survive what appears to be the theft of their future. So anger at the suffering or death of a child is a normal and justifiable process, and should be treated as such.[6]

Coping with anger

Medical staff need to lead angry parents through their anger. They can do this by:

- *listening* to the parents without interrupting

- *looking* at the parents while they are speaking

- *not attempting to justify* at this stage any action taken by the medical team; it is possibly that the anger is not misdirected. Even if, as in the story on page 165, the anger is a blind hitting out at the nearest person, justification is not appropriate at this point – it will simply exacerbate the anger

- *sympathizing* with the feeling of anger, without apportioning blame

- *never answering anger with anger.* It is important to remain warm and friendly; the anger is rarely personal, and later on, as we have seen previously, the person may be sorry, and it will have been important to have maintained a good relationship

- *being patient;* anger usually does not last. When the angry person becomes calm, the wasted energy of anger can be directed into more positive action; for example, parents can be shown how they can actively help their sick child by offering loving support and comfort – and it could be pointed out that this is something parents are better qualified to do than the medical team, for all their technical skills!

- *keeping the parents informed* – nothing makes relatives angrier than feeling that something is being kept from them

- *being quite clear* as to the wishes of the parents regarding decisions to be made

- *attempting to moderate conflict* between the parents

- *taking action* eventually by putting right misconceptions about treatment, investigating alleged errors in practice and fully explaining present policy concerning the child.

It must not be forgotten that the anger felt by the relatives of a sick child or baby may be shared by the medical team. Nurses and doctors, after months struggling to maintain the life of a fragile infant, can feel their own fury, as they see all their efforts wasted and the child sink more and more beneath the weight of his illness. This anger can also be complicated by guilt, particularly in the case of very preterm infants, or babies damaged by prolonged anoxia at time of birth who have been vigorously resuscitated. Should the medical team have made these efforts in the first place? Wouldn't it have been better to let nature take its course, rather than subject parents and child to weeks, sometimes months, of pain and anxiety, all to no avail in the end?[5] Strangely enough, in my experience the sense of futility felt in these circumstances by the caregivers is not often shared by the parents, who remain convinced that the baby should 'have his chance'. The parents' sense of futility arises from their sense that their future has been stolen from them, and they blame the medical team for failing to keep the child alive, not for saving him in the first place.

There is also a side-effect of anger:

Being angry at other people scares them away and makes it harder for them to help us.[2]

This second story shows how this can occur.

A young woman (I will call her Beth) gave premature birth to a girl child at 26 weeks gestation. Exceptionally fragile from the start, the little girl underwent long periods of ventilation. She was a great cause of anxiety to her parents and the neonatal intensive care unit (NICU) team, but she survived and went home, still requiring oxygen, after six months. In spite of her damaged lungs, the little girl was alert and bright, and everyone was proud of her. Both parents had behaved with tremendous courage throughout her stay in hospital, and there was a great sense of mutual respect and affection between parents and staff. Two months later, the little girl was readmitted with pneumonia, and a week later she was dead. Everyone grieved.

Within four months, Beth was pregnant again; the NICU team was happy for her, but doubtful of her wisdom in having another baby so soon after losing the first. The baby (a boy this time) was delivered prematurely at 28 weeks, and at first all went relatively well. Gradually, however, the little boy began to deteriorate, and after a long period of increasing weakness, in spite of all that could be done, he died; he was five months old. During this ordeal, Beth appeared a different woman. Because of her first baby, she had become used to the routine of neonatal intensive care, and she questioned every move that was made by the NICU team. She was surly with the nurses, subtly giving each to understand that she was less capable than her colleagues. She abused the doctors. She quarrelled openly with her husband; he remained loyal to her, but became increasingly silent – his own pain was never openly expressed. Beth's anger was so strong that a miasma of tension filled the NICU as soon as she entered; it became increasingly difficult to work in her presence, as she watched every move, pouncing on any action that was 'not what was done before'.

Beth was not recognizable as the courageous, caring mother who had become so attached to the staff of the NICU and continued to visit after the first baby's death. Each nurse dreaded allocation to the little boy, and, if the truth be told, could not avoid resentment at being made to feel responsible for his deterioration. In the face of such anger all doctors and nurses could do was to remain silent in the face of insult, to maintain friendship as far as was possible and, above all, to conceal their aversion from Beth, an aversion compounded by their feelings of guilt. Without being in any way to blame not only had the NICU team failed to save the two babies, but they had failed to sustain the faith and trust of the parents. An impossible situation; nothing anyone could do was right.

Everyone was filled with pity for Beth; everyone was aware of her terrible suffering yet felt helpless to alleviate it in any way. *How else but with anger could she cope with such a profound and prolonged ordeal?* The courage, the trust, the hope she had shown during the struggle for the life of the first child, she could not maintain for the second. And who could blame her? Perhaps, twice bereft in a manner so unnatural and implacable, the only way she could survive was to 'Rage, rage against the dying of the light.'

References

1   Barber H (1947) *The Occasion Fleeting.* H K Lewis, London.

2   Speck P (1978) *Loss and Grief in Medicine.* Baillière Tindall, London.

3   Kushner H S (1982) *When Bad Things Happen to Good People.* Pan Books, London.

4   Kohner N and Henley A (1991) *When a Baby Dies.* Pandora Press, London.

5   Storkey E (1989) *Losing a Child.* Lion Publishing, Oxford.

6   Sparshott M M (1996) *Pain, Distress and the Newborn Baby.* Blackwell Science, Oxford.

Dear Relatives,

We have talked in the last chapter of angry *relatives, but not for a moment do we forget that most of you were never angry – and that the rest of you were angry only occasionally and often with good cause.*

We have constantly admired:

—   *your courage when we had to give you bad news and you were seized by the terrible icy grip of fear*

—   *the way you coped with the strain of struggling to balance too much hope with too little*

—   *your patience and good humour when we kept you waiting – and then when we didn't understand, or didn't explain, as well as we should have done.*

We have shared with you not only peaks of hope and some pleasant surprises, but also troughs of setback and despair.

Frequently, we have felt how much more we could have done for you, if only we had more time.

We have learned much from you. Thank you for what you have taught us.

Further reading

General

Barber H (1947) *The Occasion Fleeting*. H K Lewis, London.

Brewin T (1996) *The Friendly Professional: selected writings of Thurstan Brewin* (ed. G Rees). Eurocommunica Publications, Bognor Regis, PO22 9RR.

Doyle D (1989) Talking to the Dying Patient. In *Talking with Patients – a Basic Clinical Skill* (ed. P R Myerscough). Oxford University Press, Oxford.

Faulkner A and Maguire P (1994) *Talking to Cancer Patients and their Relatives*. Oxford University Press, Oxford.

Kubler Ross E (1970) *On Death and Dying*. Tavistock Publications, London.

Maguire P (1994) Psychological Aspects of Breast Cancer. *BMJ*. **309**: 1649–52.

Monroe B (1993) The Psycho-social Dimension of Palliation. In *Management of Terminal Malignant Disease*, 3rd edn (eds C Saunders and N Sykes). Edward Arnold, London.

Parkes C M (1986) *Bereavement,* 2nd edn. Penguin Books, London.

Ryle J (1948) *The Natural History of Disease*. Oxford University Press, Oxford.

Wilkes E (1989) Ethics in Terminal Care. In *Doctors' Decisions* (eds G R Dunstan and E A Shinebourne). Oxford University Press, Oxford.

Chapter 1

Joyce C R B, Capble G, Mason M *et al.* (1969) Quantitative Study of Doctor–Patient Communications. *Quarterly Journal of Medicine*. **38**: 183–94.

Ley P and Llewelyn S (1995) Improving Patients' Understanding, Recall, Satisfaction and Compliance. In *Health Psychology: Processes and Applications* (eds A Broome and S Llewelyn). Chapman Hall, London.

Lipkin M (1987) The Medical Interview and Related Skills. In *Office Practice of Medicine,* 2nd edn (ed. W T Branch). W B Saunders, Philadelphia.

Chapter 4

Gould H and Toghill P J (1981) How Should We Talk about Leukaemia to Adult Patients and Their Families? *BMJ.* **282**: 210–12.

Marteau T M (1994) Psychology and Screening: Narrowing the Gap Between Efficacy and Effectiveness. *British Journal of Clinical Psychology.* **33**: 1–10.

Palmer A G, Tucker S, Warren R *et al.* (1993) Understanding Women's Responses to Treatment for Cervical Intra-epithelial Neoplasia. *British Journal of Clinical Psychology.* **32**: 101–12.

Posen S (1993) The Portrayal of the Physician in Non-medical Literature. *Journal of the Royal Society of Medicine.* **86**: 582–6.

Chapter 6

Carnwath T C M and Johnson D A W (1987) Psychiatric Morbidity Among Spouses of Patients with Stroke. *BMJ.* **294**: 409–11.

Hill A Bradford (1963) Medical Ethics and Controlled Trials. *BMJ.* **1**: 1043–9

Kerr D N and Davidson S (1958) Gastrointestinal Intolerance to Oral Iron Preparations. *Lancet.* **2**: 489–92.

Mayou R, Williamson B and Foster A (1976) Attitudes and Advice after Myocardial Infarction. *BMJ.* **2**: 1577–9.

Schwartz D and Lellouch J (1967) Explanatory and Pragmatic Attitudes in Therapeutic Trials. *Journal of Chronic Disease.* **20**: 637–48.

Stalker D and Glymour C (1989) *Examining Holistic Medicine.* Prometheus Books, New York.

Chapter 8

Hill O and Blendis L (1967) Physical and Psychological Evaluation of 'Non-organic' Abdominal Pain. *Gut.* **8**: 221–9.

Speck P (1978) *Loss and Grief in Medicine.* Baillière Tindall, London.

Chapter 10

Gilley J (1988) Intimacy and Terminal Care. *Journal of the Royal College of General Practitioners.* **38**: 121–2.

Saunders C M (1983) Terminal Care. In *Oxford Textbook of Medicine.* Oxford University Press, Oxford.

Chapter 11

Black J (1987) Broaden Your Mind about Death and Bereavement in Certain Ethnic Groups in Britain. *BMJ.* **295**: 536–9.

Buckman R (1992) *How To Break Bad News.* Papermac, London.

Chana J, Rhys-Maitland R, Hon P *et al.* (1990) Who Asks Permission for an Autopsy? *Journal of the Royal College of Physicians.* **24**: 185–8.

Charlton R (1994) Autopsy and Medical Education: A Review. *Journal of the Royal Society of Medicine.* **87**: 232–5.

Gatrad A R (1994) Muslim Customs Surrounding Death, Bereavement, Postmortem Examinations, and Organ Transplants. *BMJ.* **309**: 521–3.

Morton J B and Leonard D R A (1979) Cadaver Nephrectomy: An Operation on the Donor's Family. *BMJ.* **1**: 239–41.

Orwell G (1970) *Collected Essays, 1945–1950.* Penguin Books, London.

Stein A, Hope T and Baum J D (1995) Organ Transplantation: Approaching the Donor's Family. *BMJ.* **310**: 1149–50.

Chapter 12

Ritchie J and Davies S (1995) Professional Negligence: A Duty of Candid Disclosure? *BMJ.* **310**: 888–9.

Index